RAW FREEDOM

Combining the best of raw with healthy cooked foods for the ultimate diet

By Frederic Patenaude

Copyright information

Cover art: Martin Mailloux

Important Medical Disclaimer

The information in this book does not constitute medical or health advice, but is presented simply with the intention of sharing the personal experiences of Frederic Patenaude with healthful living.

Frederic Patenaude does not provide any medical opinions or health advice. If you have questions regarding specific medical or healthcare matters, you should speak directly with your doctor or licensed healthcare provider.

The information contained in this book is not intended to replace the advice of a licensed healthcare provider.

Raw Freedom

Acknowledgements

This work would not have been possible without the help of some dear friends who pushed me to finish it and helped me organize my thoughts in a more concise manner.

Special thanks go to Shelli Stein for helping me clarify many areas of this book.

Thanks to Kevin Gianni for helpful insights while I was working on the book.

Thanks to Ela Harrison Gordon for her editing skills and helping me finish parts of this book.

Thanks to Terry Dean for giving this book direction and focus.

Thanks to Olivier Magnan for pushing me to get it done!

Thanks to all my readers for their useful suggestions and for being the reason I wrote this book.

"Eating should be a genuine guilt-free pleasure, which must include the absence of a stressful internal dialogue."

Table of Contents

Introduction

I've wanted to write this book for many years, but never got around to doing so. I wasn't sure how to present my ideas, and more importantly, I wasn't sure how well they would be received. I think that now the time is ripe for this book, on which I've worked in one form or another since 2004.

What exactly is the premise of "Raw Freedom?"

This book is meant for you if you are:

- Considering the raw food diet lifestyle.
- Already following some kind of raw food program.
- Wanting to improve your health by adding more raw foods to your diet.

Within one of these categories, you also find:

- You're not interested in eating 100% raw, or you're fed up with it.
- You're looking for an alternative to the strict raw food diet promoted everywhere as the "holy grail" of health.
- You've experienced some health problems or failed to solve your own health problems following a raw food diet or similar programs.
- You want to eat a super-healthy diet that fits with your personality and your life, and you want to eat both raw foods and cooked foods.

This book is unlike any other book I've written because it's one that could only come from what is now almost two decades of experience in this field. This is where "the path of health" has led me.

The basic concept of this book — to offer an alternative to the rigid raw food diet — has always been the same, but it went through different forms in its development. I've actually scrapped every previous version or concept, as I felt I was not ready to release something of that nature until now.

Previous names/ideas have included:

- "The Mostly Raw Plan" — how to design a mostly raw diet that works
- "The Raw Food Dilemma" — finding the balance between raw and cooked
- "The Raw Fusion Diet — fusion of raw foods and cooked foods

I never had the guts to write the book because I felt I would be castigated and ostracized by the raw food community for doing so.

Also, my ideas were not exactly ripe. This is not a book I could have written at the age of 26. But I can at the age of 37, with enough life experience under my belt to feel confident that my words will be valuable to a lot of people.

Over the past few years, I've noticed a wind of change within the raw food community. People are openly discussing problems they had been having with the raw food diet and looking for alternatives. Even the "gurus" who previously claimed that unless you ate 100% raw you couldn't possibly get all the good results are now more lenient.

This is the right time for me to add this book to the conversation. A lot of people may not agree with it—I'm sure it will cause more of a stir than any other book I've released, but I've never felt it was more important to come out with it than I do now.

According to an article published in Medical News, the raw food diet is the second-most-popular diet at the moment, after the ever-popular Atkins program. Raw food restaurants are popping up all over North America, more and more books are being published on the subject, raw foodists are appearing on television and radio shows telling the world about their amazing recoveries from various diseases, and several companies are now selling a complete array of products tailored to people interested in the raw food lifestyle.

This book is not the typical raw food diet information book. The purpose of this book is to offer an alternative to the rigid and idealistic raw food diet presented by most other authors.

Enjoy!

Frédéric Patenaude

February 17ᵗʰ
Repentigny, Quebec, Canada

What is Raw Freedom?

This book is about creating a healthy, practical diet with a strong emphasis on raw foods, but not one that is so restrictive that it requires a 100% commitment to eating only uncooked foods.

It's a fusion/inclusion program that recognizes that eating a big percentage of raw foods provides clear benefits, but cooking certain foods does too.

It's also a way out for many raw foodists and health enthusiasts who can't seem to find a balance, and too often hover between two extremes with a lot of associated guilt, often induced by years of striving to eat a diet that is frankly too restrictive.

In this book, you'll sometimes see me refer to certain people in the raw food "world" in seemingly pejorative terms, such as the *raw food police*, raw food *fanatics,* and raw food *gurus.* This is not because I want to imply that people following a raw food diet are necessarily all deluded. I have been one of these people (policeman, fanatic and guru all at the same time!) and I also know that for many individuals, a 100% raw food diet gives them the health and balance they seek. This book is not written for those who have found such balance, but to everyone else, who may be seduced by the raw food message, but are not able to make it work the way it's supposed to work according to the books and gurus.

Yet, at the same time, due to a lack of understanding of certain physiological principles at play, and a lot of bad science used in the raw food movement, the trend is for everybody to beat themselves up for their so-called "failures" at applying a diet that is not sustainable for a large number of people to begin with. That is why I will cast light on the dark side of the raw food movement as a whole; not to imply too much negativity, but simply to make a point that needs to be made.

The program that I'm proposing in this book is flexible and easily customizable. If you can get just a few good ideas from this book that make a difference in your health and your life, I will have achieved my goal.

This book contains practical advice, not theories. Therefore, I will not spend too much time trying to debunk every single questionable statement to be heard in the health food world, or try to prove points that any honest health-seeker can easily verify by examining the scientific consensus on the topic.

This book is really more about the experience of *one* person — yours truly — both in having experimented with raw food and vegan lifestyles for more than 15 years, but also in having worked with thousands of people through a website that receives more than 70,000 unique visitors a month, and in person at numerous events I've attended over the years. I feel I have a good grasp of the realities faced by the outside-of-the-box individuals who find themselves attracted to vegetarianism, veganism and raw foodism — but I also want to repeat that my experience is subjective. I invite you to view what I say not with skepticism, but with an open mind. More importantly, I invite you to trust *yourself* and your own experience. If what I share with you strikes a familiar chord, then use the information for your benefit. If it doesn't, just move on.

Inclusion vs. Exclusion

What all diet books have in common is that they all tell you what you should *not* be eating. Each diet needs a *villain* that's universally responsible for all your ills. Raw foodists blame cooked foods. Paleo diets blame carbs. The new *Wheat Belly* fad blames wheat. Vegans blame animal products in all their forms. Plant-based advocates and natural hygienists blame oil and fat.

The easier and more identifiable the target is, the more simplistic the program will be. And simplicity helps sell books. The problem is that there's nothing simplistic about the human body and the complex processes involved in human nutrition. In fact, as far as we know, the human body (and brain) could be the most complex organism in the universe.

So to blame all diet-related health problems on *one* factor would be missing the mark in a major way, especially when we consider the obvious:–

If cooked foods were truly the cause of most human illnesses, then how come all the longest lived people eat cooked foods, including almost all known centenarians? And how come not a single culture on the planet has ever eaten an exclusively raw food diet?

If grains were truly the cause of the "obesity epidemic" in what is often dubbed a *carb-crazed nation*, then how come billions of people have done just fine for millennia eating a rice-based diet, and stayed very trim and healthy eating outrageous amounts of carbs?

If carbs were truly the problem, then all come all the longest lived cultures in the world eat carbs? And how come the human body seems to be *designed* to enjoy carbs, with the sweet taste sensation being the most prominent feature of our sensory system for recognizing food?

If fat was truly the problem, then how come mother's milk is over 50% fat by calories. And if sugar was really the problem, again, how come mother's milk is over 40% sugar by calories?

Behind every health craze, there's some truth. The mistake is to believe in a one-sided answer that, in light of the complexities of the systems that regulate our health, can frankly be seriously flawed.

So for a change, this book will focus more on *inclusion* rather than *exclusion*.

I won't tell you that the key to this program is to eliminate entire categories of food from your diet. I'll try to put things in perspective, and let you make your own choices based on your own preferences and knowledge of your own body.

So consider *Raw Freedom* a "fusion-inclusion" program that combines the best of raw foods with really healthy cooked foods, to create a sustainable diet that even gives you some leeway in making your own decisions.

The Main Advantages of Raw Foods

The idea behind *Raw Freedom* is to recognize that certain benefits can be derived from eating raw foods, but without restricting oneself to *only* raw foods. We need to take a look at the health advantages that can be obtained from a raw food diet, and then ask which of those benefits come from eating raw foods exclusively, and which could be attained in a less restrictive manner.

A raw food diet, or something close to it, has huge advantages. Otherwise, nobody would do it. Let's take a good look at what the benefits are, but also understand where these benefits come from. Once we are clear about the benefits and what creates them in the raw food diet specifically, we can design our *raw freedom* approach that combines the best from both raw and cooked worlds.

Easy weight management

This topic will be extensively covered in later parts of this book. For now, let's just summarize the obvious: it's extremely difficult to gain weight eating only raw fruits and vegetables. There are two reasons for this. The first is that fruits and vegetables have an extremely low caloric density. Meaning, that by weight, they contain fewer calories than most other foods. One pound of raw vegetables contains on average 100 calories. One pound of fruit contains 250 calories on average. On the other hand, one pound of bread contains 1500 calories and one pound of lean meat still contains close to 900 calories. The second reason is that the calories in raw foods are less "accessible" than calories in cooked foods. Recent research has demonstrated this.[1] Cooking pre-digests many foods, even fruit, making the foods more calorie dense. On average, I've found that raw foods contain 15-20% fewer calories than listed values. All of these factors combined make it extremely difficult for anyone to gain weight,

---

1   See book "Catching Fire" and documentary "Did Cooking Make Us Humans"

and in fact not *lose* weight, eating only raw foods, unless one includes in larger quantities the few caloric-dense foods that a raw food diet generally allows, such as nuts, seeds, avocados and, to some degree, oils.

Caloric Density

One of the most important concepts to understand in human nutrition is that of caloric density. Caloric density is the proportion of a food's energy content to its weight.

For example, an entire head of lettuce weighing over one pound contains less than 100 calories. This means that the caloric density of lettuce is less than 100 calories per pound.

On the other hand, one single tablespoon of oil contains 120 calories. So you have more calories in one tablespoon of oil than in a pound of lettuce. But guess which is going to fill you up more?

You can use the concept of caloric density when you make food choices so that you fill up on foods that have a lot of volume, but few calories by weight. Eating these foods, you'll feel satisfied and full, and will be able to eat as much as you want, and may even lose weight in the process.

Studies have confirmed that if you feed people foods of low caloric density, they will eat as much as they want, not be hungry, and lose weight, without having to count calories.

Because these foods have so few calories, it's almost impossible to create a caloric excess eating them.

Let's take a look at the average caloric density of certain foods. Keep in mind that this is an average across a category. For example, we know that bananas contain more calories by weight than apples, but overall, members of any category have similar caloric density.

Food	Caloric Density Per Pound
Fresh Raw or Cooked Veggies	100
Fresh Raw Fruit	250-300
Cooked Starchy Vegetables	450-500
Intact Whole Grains	450-500
Legumes and Beans	550-600
Meat Products	900-1000
Dried Fruit	1200
Processed Grains and Flours	1200-1500
Cheese	1800
Nuts and Seeds	2800
Oil	4000

Looking at this table, you might be tempted to only eat vegetables, as they contain only 100 calories per pound. It's important to note that nobody can live on just vegetables, and that you'd get so hungry on a diet of just vegetables, you'd eventually break down and eat something else!

However, you want your diet to contain plenty of raw vegetables by weight.

The point is to look at the overall caloric density of your meals each day.

Experiments have shown that people will lose weight if the caloric density of their food is less than 400 calories per pound. That is eating as much as they want and without exercise.

The reason why the raw food diet is so effective for weight loss is because of its low caloric density. Athletes, who need more calories, can get them by blending fruits, increasing their caloric density by breaking down the fiber and reducing the volume.

Low-toxin diet

A raw vegan diet is an extremely low-toxin diet. Raw fruits and vegetables are digested almost effortlessly and contribute very little stress to the body. They are also less allergenic than other foods, such as wheat. Concentrations of pesticides, heavy metals and other measurable toxins are quite low in fresh produce, compared to animal products. Raw fruits and vegetables are also very alkaline-forming after digestion. Also, the raw food diet *excludes* a lot of foods that are potentially carcinogenic: grilled meats, baked carbohydrates, refined and factory-made foods, food preservatives, dairy products, etc. In addition to avoidance of all these carcinogens, fruits and vegetables—as well as nuts and seeds—contain powerful antioxidants that prevent cancer. Therefore a raw food diet can be extremely effective in the prevention of cancer, as well as other degenerative diseases, such as heart disease. Raw foodists rarely suffer from these problems. In fact, diseases of excess are rarely an issue in individuals following a raw food diet. Common problems are more related to deficiencies rather than excess.

Nutrient Density

Fruits and vegetables are the most nutrient dense foods on the planet. When we say that a food is "nutrient dense," we mean it has a high concentration of nutrients (such as vitamins and minerals) per calorie. Starchy foods are *calorie* dense, but not as *nutrient* dense as fruits and vegetables.

In other words, 500 calories of rice or potatoes will contain fewer vitamins, minerals, and phytochemicals than 500 calories of kale or 500 calories of apple.

By eating a diet composed mainly of raw fruits and vegetables, we take in more nutrients for fewer calories than if we were to eat mostly cooked grains and meat, or even cooked starchy vegetables.

There are some exceptions, however. Cooked greens tend to be more nutrient dense than raw greens, simply because they wilt down and we can eat more of them that way.

For example, you've probably taken a huge amount of spinach and cooked it down to almost nothing in a matter of seconds. Well, that small cup of cooked spinach is now jam-packed with the minerals of the huge amount of raw spinach, and will only take you a few minutes to eat. On the other hand, the raw spinach takes much longer to chew. Therefore, cooked spinach is more nutrient dense than raw spinach because we can eat more of it more easily.

Raw foodists can get around this by blending greens. Thanks to blenders, we can make a huge green smoothie that will contain a good amount of spinach or kale, and drink it down in no time. It goes without saying that having some form of processed greens in the diet, whether they are steamed or blended, is essential for getting a good balance of nutrients.

Certain cooked foods are as nutrient dense as raw foods, but the most nutrient dense foods are still fruits and vegetables, whether raw or cooked. For example, cooked sweet potato is very nutrient dense, but the same cannot be said of cooked white pasta.

By getting enough calories from raw fruits and vegetables, we automatically take in more than enough vitamins, minerals, and other essential and protective nutrients. This is one of the main reasons why the raw food diet can be effective.

Phytochemicals

Raw fruits and vegetables, as well as raw nuts and seeds, are packed with phytochemicals.

"Phyto" means "plant," so the term *phytochemical* designates different compounds in plant foods that protect against illness. Some phytochemicals can prevent DNA damage caused by free radicals.

You've probably heard that antioxidants with cancer-preventing benefits are found in many fruits and vegetables and dark leafy greens. Antioxidants are a class of phytochemicals. Some of the most potent phytochemicals are found in raw foods, and many of them are heat-sensitive. Therefore, eating a raw food diet or a mostly raw diet will give you an abundance of phytochemicals — and this could prove to be one of the main benefits of the diet.

Some notable phytochemicals are to be found in:

#1: The cruciferous family. Including cabbage, kale, broccoli, etc. These vegetables contain a class of phytochemicals (called sulphoraphane and indole-3-carbinol) that are converted into cancer-fighting enzymes by the liver, and also help to balance estrogen levels.

#2: Berries. Including pomegranates, cherries, blueberries, grapes, etc. They contain many phytochemicals that increase immunity.

#3: Citrus fruits. Close to their skin, these fruits contain many phytochemicals, in addition to lots of vitamin C, which is an antioxidant.

Every raw fruit and vegetable contains health-enhancing phytochemicals. Cooking food sometimes enhances the bioavailability of certain phytochemicals, like lycopene in tomatoes, but many antioxidants are more available in the raw state.

Low Toxic Load

A compound called acrylamide is created when carbohydrates (such as potatoes) are cooked at high temperatures (as in baking, frying, etc.). In animal studies, high doses of acrylamide have been shown to cause cancer. More acrylamide is created when foods are cooked at higher temperatures or for longer periods of time.

We also know that other molecules, called "Maillard Molecules," are formed when foods brown and caramelize during cooking. Some people speculate that these new compounds, created in the cooking process, may affect health negatively.

While certain forms of cooking appear to be relatively harmless (steaming, for example), the surest way to reduce the amount of toxins in your diet is to eat some foods in their raw state.

Note that sometimes cooking destroys toxins that are naturally present in plants. So it's important to avoid certain foods that should never be eaten raw, like raw or sprouted legumes. For more foods that should never be eaten raw, please consult my book *Raw Food Controversies*.

Increased immunity

For the reasons listed above, a raw food diet can be a very effective tool in boosting natural immunity. It's not the fact that foods are eaten *raw* that makes such a difference, but rather that fruits and vegetables (whether raw or cooked) contain plenty of antioxidants that boost immunity. Also, many foods and substances that can weaken immunity are generally excluded on a raw food diet.

Eliminating Everything Else That's Bad for You

One of the main reasons people get sick is that they eat so many "dead," pre-packaged foods. These foods are not only heavily processed, but contain a long list of suspicious ingredients, including MSG, preservatives, artificial coloring, and more.

Eating a raw food diet automatically eliminates all of this junk, which means your diet will be 100% more clean and pure. It will be "wholesome" in the true sense of the world, not the adulterated sense misused everywhere in food advertising.

The raw food diet also generally avoids grains, a category of food many people have allergic reactions to (especially the gluten-containing grains).

False Science Used by Raw Foodists to Promote Their Diet

Over the years, I've evolved from a very idealistic, somewhat naive view of raw food nutrition, based on the radical energy of my early twenties, to a more mature and complete understanding of the whole picture today.

The problem is that most people starting out on the raw food diet are still hanging on to misinformation, and receive bad advice from raw food authors that is not based in science, but rather in what I call "raw food lore."

In the end, the raw food diet may very well provide great benefits, but not for the reasons raw foodists claim. Let's review the most glaring pieces of misinformation that are common in raw food circles and that make this diet the laughingstock of the scientific community.

Remember, the fact that all these "facts" are completely false does not undermine the actual benefits of the diet. Rather, it can mislead raw foodists into making choices that are less than excellent. It also undermines the credibility of the movement, which is often seen as more of a circus of clowns than a true health movement.

#1: "Cooking destroys digestive enzymes."

By far the biggest raw food myth is that of digestive enzymes. I remember when I first got into raw foods, I was told that cooking anything above 115 degrees Fahrenheit destroyed those living enzymes, and that's why we get sick. I believed it, even though there wasn't a shred of true science behind it.

The reality is that although plant enzymes exist, they are made for the survival of the plant itself. For example, enzymes in bananas transform the starch in a green banana into sugar as it ripens. Those enzymes are not necessary for humans, as we produce our own enzymes to digest food.

Even if you could somehow prove that food enzymes are beneficial when isolated, those same enzymes in foods are denatured and deactivated as soon as they reach our stomach. They can't resist the high acidity of the human stomach.

It's also false to believe that the human body has a limited supply of enzymes that "runs out" as it gets older. This ludicrous idea was propagated by the mysterious "doctor" Howell, who wrote a famous book on enzymes, which, by the way, has no real scientific references to support any of its claims.

Enzymes are also not alive. They are just proteins that catalyze chemical reactions which could not take place without their presence. Enzymes can only work under very specific conditions, such as the right temperature, pH, and the presence of other co-enzymes. Plant enzymes themselves will only work under a different set of parameters than our own digestive enzymes, which ultimately renders them useless after we eat them.

#2: "Fruits and vegetables are the human-specific diet"

The raw food diet is often promoted based on the idea that humans once lived on a pure raw food diet in perfect health, and as they discovered cooking, and eventually agriculture, their health began to deteriorate, culminating in the current state of bad health people experience today.

Every single discovery in the study of human evolution disproves this fantasy.

First of all, there is credible evidence that humans have been cooking for a very long time. A recent discovery[2] showed that the extinct early hominid species *homo erectus* was cooking food, which would place cooking as beginning over 1.9 million years ago.

It's true that *homo erectus* did not evolve into *homo sapiens*, but is an extinct cousin family. However, the research shows that cooking is much more ancient than we originally believed.

Researcher Professor Richard Wrangham argues in his book *Catching Fire* that cooking food enabled humans to evolve. Why? Because it enabled us to get more calories and not spend 60-75% of our time looking for food and chewing it, like other apes.

Our digestive system even adapted to this change by becoming shorter, allowing for much quicker digestion than in other apes and removing the ability to extract much nutrition from insoluble fiber, much of which is already broken down by cooking.

Cooking gave humans an unmatched advantage by making available calorie denser storable foods that could not be consumed otherwise (like tubers), thus allowing for year-round food in a single place.

Modern raw foodists also eat a diet that is nowhere close to that of other apes. We do our own version of cooking and processing with blenders, dehydrators, and other modern appliances, making fibrous vegetables, and even fruit, easier to digest.

#3: "Humans are the only species who cook their food and the only species who suffer from degenerative diseases!"

I never fully believed the myth that wild animals don't suffer from disease, but it is still a commonly seen argument for a raw food diet.

---

2   http://www.guardian.co.uk/science/2011/aug/22/cooking-origins-homo-erectus)

Wild animals do suffer from a wide range of diseases, but typically some of these could be avoided in the context of modern medicine. In other words, deaths by parasites and infectious disease are common.

Generally, it is true that wild animals don't suffer from common degenerative diseases that affect humans, such as heart disease. However, wild animals do die of various kinds of cancer, even if they don't live in polluted areas.

The problem with this argument is that although it contains a grain of truth, it leads one to believe that a raw food diet is the only way to perfect health. Raw foodists do die from diseases, and in some cases those diseases have nothing to do with their diet (or could not be improved through dietary changes alone). Raw foodists have a lifespan that is quite average in general. This is not something that has been scientifically proven, but a personal observation of mine. If most raw foodists reached a very advanced age, I would have heard about it by now.

I would avoid the "wild animals" argument, because humans are so different from wild animals in so many ways that we can't possibly compare ourselves to them anyway.

Wild animals don't wear clothes... Should we try not to either?

#4: "Cooking food turns it into poison."

Cooking food does affect it at the molecular level. In some cases, raw foods that contain real poisons are rendered edible by cooking. For example, raw kidney beans are poisonous, but by soaking and cooking them we destroy the enzyme inhibitors that can cause serious food poisoning if those beans are eaten raw.

On the other hand, cook some steak over the grill, and you'll create a series of new, carcinogenic compounds that were not present in the steak before, and we saw a few pages ago that acrylamide, produced by high-heat cooking of carbohydrates, is carcinogenic.

On the other hand, certain methods of cooking, such as steaming, appear rather innocuous. Of course, raw foodists will say that we don't know yet what possible toxic compounds are created in any form of cooking, so steamed broccoli could be just as bad as barbecued meat, just for different reasons. This is, of course, pure conjecture, and most likely not true.

If cooked food were truly toxic, the human race would have disappeared a long time ago. This argument doesn't do a lot of good for the credibility of the raw food movement.

#5: "Cooking destroys the natural live energy in food."

Some raw foodists have used the "vital energy" argument to promote a raw food diet. The idea is that raw foods contain some kind of vital force that is destroyed by cooking.

To prove their point, they will show you Kirlian photographs (a special type of photography that captures a sort of "aura" around an object), showing the difference between raw and cooked foods. Raw foods appear bright with a beautiful aura, while the aura of the same foods when cooked appears dead, with depressing colors.

Kirlian photography uses a high-voltage source connected to a photographic plate. The object being photographed will be in contact with the plate. Because low current electricity is used, the technique is harmless.

According to Media College:

> Small coronal discharges are created by the strong electric field at the edges of the object. The frequency of the electricity excites electrons in the object so they ionize the surrounding air.

> Objects must be conductive for this technique to work. The object can be moist (e.g. a living thing), or conduct metal. A dry non-conducting object will not produce the effect. (...)

Many paranormal enthusiasts still claim that the aura captured by Kirlian photography is some sort of "life force."

However this is easily debunked:

#1: Kirlian photographs can be taken of anything moist or conductive, including coins, paperclips, etc.

#2: Kirlian photographs taken in a vacuum (where no ionized gas is present) show no aura.

#3: Some people claim that a living object slowly loses its aura after it dies. This is more easily explained by the fact that it loses its moisture.

Because raw foods have a high moisture content, they appear more vibrant under Kirlian photography than their cooked counterparts.

#6: "Raw foods are easier to digest than cooked foods."

It is true that some raw foods are much easier to digest than some cooked foods, but in most cases this is not true.

One example: starchy foods are easier to digest cooked than raw. This category includes potatoes, rice, and pretty much all grains. No population could ever survive eating these foods raw, as we only digest a tiny percentage of the raw starch, compared to most of the cooked starch. Raw starch probably won't harm you, but you just can't digest much of it.

Most of the world's population lives on a starch-based diet, because it is simply a more reliable source of calories.

When raw foodists try to take some grains or beans and eat them raw, I always laugh. I've seen recipes that called for soaking rice to "sprout" it, and then turning it into a dish. But raw rice, even when soaked and sprouted, has very little nutritional value, because we don't digest most of what's in it. At least raw rice is not toxic, unlike many kinds of beans that can put you in the hospital if you eat them raw (such as kidney beans).

How to Strengthen Your Digestion and Avoid the Most Common Problems of Restricted Diets: Intolerance

This is a dilemma that every person who has seriously dabbled with raw foodism, fasting, juice cleansing and even other restricted diets — has experienced. When one has lived on a restricted diet for a good period of time, reintroduction of previously perfectly digestible foods will cause extreme symptoms of indigestion and sickness. It happens to raw foodists. It happens to "low-carb" and "no-carb" dieters. It happens to those who eliminate gluten completely, believing they are intolerant (when often it is not the case). It happens to those addicted to water fasting, juice "feasts," and other forms of cleansing. It also happens to those who try to follow calorie-restricted diets, or no-salt diets.

The more restricted the diet is, the more difficult the reintroduction of other foods will be. Water fasting, which involves the temporary elimination of ALL sources of nourishment except water and the body's own reserves, weakens the digestion so much that refeeding after a fast is extremely delicate. Improper refeeding after a long fast can even lead to death, as it has been the case in a few people who ate too enthusiastically after a long fast.

After the 23-day water fast I undertook in Costa Rica in 2005, I had digestive disorders and could only properly digest small quantities of fruits and vegetables. However, my body needed a lot more than a few fruits. But eating large fruit meals that were served at the fasting retreat caused painful and urgent bowel movements. It literally took months for my digestion to return to normal after the fast.

The weakening of digestive power after a long fast is understandable, as the body has not practiced digesting anything for days and weeks. Retraining it takes time and patience, and most importantly, careful monitoring.

Restricted diets also significantly lower digestive power, and make people sick when they "fall off the wagon" and occasionally cheat. This is actually the biggest reason people "feel like crap" when they eat a 100% raw diet but then later reintroduce some cooked foods.

At the extreme end, a pure fruitarian diet (eating only fruits; no vegetables, no fat) would weaken digestion the most, because fruits are very simple foods composed mostly of simple sugars, very low amounts of protein, almost no fats, and fiber. Therefore, the digestion of fruits is effortless for the body.

A pure fruitarian would find it very difficult to cheat on his diet, especially if he has been following it for quite some time.

A low-fat raw foodist is not too far from a fruitarian if he follows this diet 100%. Fruits are the main source of calories, fats (which require the most digestion in this diet) are kept to a minimum, and vegetables are easy to digest. There is no starch intake, and protein is very low. Eliminating salt completely also creates other physiological adaptation, and reintroduction of foods containing salt will quickly create symptoms.

Other raw foodists who are not as strict may include some salt in their diet, perhaps some oil, and more nuts and seeds. Going off the wagon will still cause them to feel sick, although not as much so as stricter raw foodists.

What Happens When Raw Foodists Cheat

Many raw foodists have experienced extreme symptoms when going back to cooked foods. Some have even called it the "raw curse." On most other diets, being able to occasionally "cheat" or allow oneself a little reward is part of the process. Your normal diet may be strict, but on occasion you can let go a little bit. For example, someone may avoid desserts most of the time, but have a piece of cake on their birthdays.

Such flexibility makes dieting feasible. It also makes life possible. If you're invited somewhere, you can loosen your standards a bit if you like, and enjoy the company of friends, but then go back to your regular routine the next day.

Raw foodists, fruitarians, extreme dieters, and adepts of detox diets find themselves with a difficult conundrum. They may love the results they get from their raw food diet, but they also find it difficult to maintain. They crave or miss other foods, and find themselves excluded from many social interactions that are just part of life.

To most raw foodists, being able to eat raw most of the time but occasionally eat cooked foods would be ideal. However, because of their weakened digestion, whenever they "cheat" on their diet, they feel extremely sick.

And the stricter the raw food diet is, the more extreme their body's reaction will be after reintroducing cooked foods.

Here's an example I found interesting. Steve Pavlina is a well-known blogger in the sphere of personal development. He's also known for his commitment to a vegan diet, and his occasional eccentric experiments or "challenges."

As part of a series of articles for his website, he decided to give the raw food diet a try for 30 days. But he didn't just follow a regular raw food diet. He decided to go natural, and only eat raw fruits, vegetables, and minimal quantities of fat (less than 10% by total calories). He excluded all salts, spices, garlic, onion, oils, and seasonings.

He had good results in his 30-day experiment, even though he found it hard to maintain his diet. And at the end, he was looking forward to eating some cooked food.

But his first cooked meal made him extremely sick. Here's his account.

"I decided to dive right in with a cooked meal of sautéed tofu. It's a 14oz block of organic firm tofu with some tamari. I didn't use oil. The tofu has about 16g of fat. I ate it with some hot sauce (pictured) and a little vegan sour cream (not pictured). The sour cream probably added about 7–8g of fat. The whole meal is about 400 calories, about half of which are from fat.

The last time I ate cooked food after going raw for a while, it tasted totally dead to me. This time that wasn't the case at all. In fact, this food tasted better than ever. It was different than I remembered though. The tofu was so incredibly rich and creamy, and there were subtleties in the flavors I never noticed before. On the downside the hot sauce was overwhelming. Before the raw trial, I'd normally eat this with several tablespoons of hot sauce, about double the amount shown in the photo. But this time I could only finish about 80% of the hot sauce on the plate. It was so spicy, and I was sweating after just a few bites. I'd usually have this meal with about 12oz water, but this time I needed double that to stop my mouth from burning. Apparently I've lost most of my spice tolerance.

I used the same amount of tamari I used to (about 2 teaspoons). I wondered if the food would taste too salty since I haven't had any salt for 30 days. It didn't. It actually tasted less salty than I remembered, perhaps because I was focused on the creaminess and spiciness instead.

The tofu tasted so rich that it was almost like eating cheesecake. In retrospect I would have preferred half as much tofu with a large side of steamed broccoli.

Even though my stomach felt full afterwards, I had the urge to scarf down at least another pound of food or a green smoothie. It felt odd to stop eating so soon.

Shortly after breakfast I felt a little loopy, almost like I'd had a couple glasses of wine. I swear my vision got a little blurry too. Those feelings passed after about 10 minutes, and then I felt very energetic and happy, almost euphoric. But I noticed my mind seemed cloudier than usual, as if a fog had just come down.

(. . .) Later this morning I had a couple slices of sprouted whole grain toast (Ezekiel 4:9 bread) with a little soy margarine. Again, it tasted better than I remembered. The flavors were so rich that it was like eating fresh baked bread right from the oven. The earthy flavors and textures seemed just perfect. It tasted so good that I ate two more slices right afterwards.

(. . .)

About an hour after eating the toast, I started feeling poorly. The first thing I noticed was that I was becoming very drowsy. I started sneezing a lot, and my nose was filling up. I didn't have any stomach problems, but I felt like I was having some kind of allergic reaction. I didn't want a complicated lunch, so I just ate 5 clementines (raw) and some pistachios (not raw).

Afternoon

A couple hours after lunch, I felt even worse, like I was coming down with a cold. I tried to nap for 90 minutes, although I probably only slept for 20. When I got up I had a mild sore throat, which I still have now.

Everyone else in my family has been sick lately, so I thought to myself, Crap. . . this is no good.

For the rest of the afternoon, I ate two green smoothies (one liter each, same kind I've been making for a while) and a Fuji apple. I started feeling a little better around 5pm but still under the weather.

For dinner I decided to brave some cooked food again, but I opted to steer clear of bread and tofu. I stir-fried some veggies (green pepper, zucchini, garlic, onion in 2 tsp olive oil), put them on a bed of steamed brown rice, and sprinkled some raw sesame seeds on top. It tasted good but no better than I expected. I ate all the veggies but didn't finish all the rice.

Later in the evening, I started feeling worse again, which is where I am now as I type this. I keep having to blow my nose, I feel a lot of tension in my neck and shoulders, I have a mild headache, and my eyes are burning a little. I took my temperature at 8:15pm, and it was 99.5. Yesterday it was 98.2.

(. . .)

I was feeling poorly with a mild fever by the end of the day. I could barely sleep at all that night, and the next day my fever spiked to 103.2. I felt totally dilapidated and nauseous and stayed in bed most of the day. (. . .)

The next day (Feb 2nd) I felt a little better. My fever dropped but was still over 100. I also had headaches cutting in and out. I ate mostly raw fruit that day, but it wasn't much because I had no appetite. I was constantly thirsty and drank many glasses of water, but it didn't quench my thirst as well as the fruit did.

(. . .)

Last night my fever finally broke, and my temperature is back down to 98.8. I have a mild sore throat.

(. . .)

It's been 3 days since I ate a cooked meal that included less than one clove of garlic, and my body still reeks of it. I woke up this morning covered in garlic sweat and tasting garlic breath. I couldn't stand the stench of myself and quickly hopped in the shower. Even after a light all-fruit breakfast, I can still taste garlic on my breath.

I gained a pound after my cooked food day, but due to this illness, I lost 5 pounds back, so I'm down another 4 pounds from the end of my original 30-day trial, 12 pounds since the start of the year. Some of that is probably due to dehydration and having very little food in me.

(. . .)

It's not at all uncommon for people to have a negative reaction to cooked food after going raw for a while. I thought it wouldn't happen to me because this was my 5th raw trial, and I never had such problems in the past when I returned to cooked food. But on my previous trials, I was including a lot more fat, dried fruits, dehydrated foods, onions, garlic, spices, hot peppers, oils, and other items I cut out for this recent trial. That seems to have made a big difference.

I find myself much less attracted to cooked food now vs. a week ago. I feel very drawn to keep eating fresh fruit. I'm actually a little turned off by bananas and attracted to juicier fruits like grapes, watermelon, Asian pears, cherries, and berries. Bananas seem too dry and pasty right now unless I blend them into a smoothie. Maybe it's because I'm dehydrated from the fever. I notice the juicy fruits quench my thirst in ways that no amount of water can. I can down a large glass of water, and I'm still thirsty a minute later. But when I eat some juicy fruit, the thirst is finally satisfied.

--

Steve's example, I think, is typical of how extreme raw foodists' reactions to normal foods can be, especially when these are reintroduced quickly after a long period of eating a very simplified diet.

A few things in his testimony stand out:

- **The tofu portion**. Steve had a *huge* portion of tofu by almost any standards. 14 ounces of tofu is a lot of tofu. Raw foodists, because they train their body to eat very large quantities of fruits and vegetables to get their calories, have actually habituated their bodies and their minds to large volumes of food. It's very difficult for an ex-raw foodist to understand what a "normal" amount of food is. For example, two ounces of tofu is a normal amount, about what Asians eat with their meals. Steve ate seven times that amount.

- **After a long period without salt and spices, the body needs some gradual readjusting if they are reintroduced**. Steve went right in and ate soy sauce and hot sauce! Not a good idea.

- **The refeeding orgy went on for the rest of the day, with lots of other cooked foods his body simply wasn't ready to digest, especially not in the quantities he tried to eat**. After a long period of time eating no oil and almost no fat, he also had two tablespoons of oil (in addition to the other fat contained in the food that day), and more seasonings (garlic, salt, etc.).

- **After being used to very juicy foods for a long period of time, his body got extremely dehydrated after eating salt**. Again, the body really adapts to foods it's given. A salt-free diet will lead to important physiological adaptations that take time to reverse. Sodium is something your body needs and salt concentration in the blood must be kept constant. If you do not take in enough salt, your body will drastically reduce its excretion of salt via urine and sweat. Then when salt is suddenly reintroduced, it increases secretion of water in order to maintain blood salt concentration and you get dehydrated. A quick change in salt intake can cause muscle cramps or weakness, or dizziness and exhaustion. But reintroducing salt after a long period of complete abstinence will also create symptoms of extreme dehydration, headaches, and more.

Steve's experiment also reminds me of an experiment I did back in 2009.

I set myself the goal of eating a pure 100% raw food diet, with no salt, no seasonings and very little fat, almost exactly what Steve Pavlina did. I was familiar with this diet of course, and I was already following it at a maybe 60 or 75% level. But I decided to go 100% for 60 days in a row.

Toward the end of my experiment, I went on a trip to Thailand, where I met up with a group of raw foodists to do some cycling.

I continued my raw food experiment and took it to around 75 days. After that point, I got stuck on an island where I did not know where fruit was sold. So I decided to end my experiment with a couple bowls of Thai soup from a street vendor, without the meat but with some cooked yuka (a tropical root).

The next day, I had a little bit of vegetarian Pad Thai when going on a diving trip (less than a cup). I also had a few pieces of a Thai dessert consisting of coconut flakes mixed with cane juice and boiled together.

That night, I slept extremely badly. The salt and spices in the food made me sweat and feel dehydrated, and I was very uncomfortable. The next day, I met with my friends and we went on an all-day biking trip in hot sun. I felt unwell but pushed myself to keep up. That day, I should have taken it easy, but I ate the most delicious durian (a unique spiky tropical fruit grown in Thailand and elsewhere in the tropics) of my life, and the next day got convinced by my friends to go on yet another biking trip.

After that day, I felt feverish. I felt pretty sick, and I knew that I could not eat more cooked food in that state, because my body had not yet adapted to it. So I spent the last week of the trip mostly in bed in my hotel room, eating only very small quantities of fruit, trying to feel better. I only felt better toward the end of my trip, when it was time to leave.

My trip to Thailand was about three weeks long, and I wasted half of it feeling sick and unable to do anything. Upon my return, I slowly and carefully reintroduced cooked foods into my diet and was able to digest them without problems.

Now some people might say that I got sick because I went on a biking trip and experienced heat exhaustion.

That's part of the answer, but what really weakened my body was eating some Thai food after two and a half months of eating a salt-free, almost fat-free raw food diet. Then cycling in the heat didn't help on top of that.

I know exactly what happened because I've heard the same story from many raw foodists from around the world who have had a similar experience.

My main regret was that I did not get to enjoy the trip to Thailand. I wanted to go there and eat great fruit, but also to experience the culture and not spend half of my time feeling sick. I should have stopped my raw food experiment before the trip and strengthened my digestion before going. The alternative would have been to stay 100% raw the whole time — something that I no longer enjoy doing when traveling.

What happens physiologically to raw foodists after long periods of time on the diet

On a raw food diet, a few things happen at the physiological level that explain the extreme reactions people get when reintroducing other foods.

Stomach stretching

The raw food diet, especially the fruit-based version, is a high-volume diet. In fact, the number one problem in newbies trying to make such a diet work is the inability to consume enough calories to sustain themselves during the day. This occurs because fruits and vegetables have a very low caloric density. As we've seen, that means significantly more volume must be consumed.

The body adapts to the caloric density of a diet by stretching its stomach to allow larger volumes of food to be digested. Author Dr. Doug Graham, who advocates a low-fat, high-fruit, raw vegan diet, recommends going on a sort of "stomach stretching" program to handle the large quantities of food that are required to maintain this diet.

> "It takes some practice to develop the ability to consume what, from the raw perspective, should be thought of as "normal" amounts of food for a human. Somewhere in between "all you care for" and "all you can" there is a happy medium that will enable you to increase the amount you consume. The stomach is very accommodating in this regard and will stretch quickly to allow you to consume normal/healthy quantities of fruit. At the same time, your image of what is a healthy amount, and your mindset about quantities of fruit will grow to match your ability to eat it." If you practice eating a meal of just fruit, only fruit, and nothing but fruit, it will get easier and easier to consume appropriate volumes.[3]

---

3   http://foodnsport.com/faq.php

Psychologically, the mind also gets used to very large meals as a routine.

When describing the raw food diet as high-volume, I am not saying that it is worse because more volume is consumed. In fact, the low caloric density of fruits and vegetables is an advantage that certainly helps the dieter and allows for easy maintenance of one's body weight. Because it is more *difficult* to get enough calories from fruits and vegetables, it is also more *difficult* to gain weight on such a diet.

However, eating a 100% raw food diet, especially one that excludes all concentrated foods (oils, large quantities of nuts, dried fruits, etc.) requires ever-larger quantities of food for maintaining this diet in the long term.

In the first few months, most people will lose weight on a raw diet and will be happy about the results. However, when ideal weight is reached, the deficit in calories can no longer be maintained. That means that most people wanting to follow this type of diet for long periods of time must eventually train their bodies to consume a greater volume of food.

There is also another factor that explains why raw foodists have difficulties getting enough calories from their diet, and that's the digestibility of calories. We tend to think of calories as just units of energy in food, which are calculated by scientists and are absolute, regardless of how the foods are prepared.

If a raw carrot has 50 calories, then a cooked carrot also has 50 calories, right? If a raw banana has 100 calories, then a cooked banana must be the same?

New research shows that raw foods are less digestible than cooked foods, meaning that there are fewer calories available in raw foods. I've noticed that fact for a long time, but there was little science to back it up.

One clear observation is that raw foodists following a diet that *excludes* all refined and concentrated foods (such as oils), require 15-20% more calories for the same level of calories. So a man that normally needs 3000 calories on a normal diet would require around 3500 calories on a low fat raw vegan diet. A woman needing 2000 calories on a cooked diet would need 2300 to 2400 calories on a raw diet.

On the one hand, the ideal raw food diet is composed of fruits, vegetables, and small quantities of fatty foods. This diet also has a low caloric density (because fruits and vegetables have fewer calories per pound than other foods), but also because food is eaten 100% raw (as opposed to cooked), the average person following this program will need an extra 15-20% calories to maintain their body weight.

All of this to say that a LOT of volume must be consumed. How much volume?

Now that raw foodists from around the world can share on the Internet in Ning forums, ideas can be exchanged really fast. The concept that *it takes more food than you think to make this diet work* has caught on with anyone serious enough about this lifestyle. One raw foodist writes:

> I was having a lot of trouble with this diet until I started eating 4500+ calories per day from RIPE fruit. Veggies are good, but you should skip them if you're under-carbed or trying to train / expand your stomach. Nuts or dried fruit have zero appeal to me unless I'm significantly under-fed... don't even get me started on cooked food or animal products... no need for that... ever...

> I often eat 22 un-blended bananas before 11 AM ... You say you can't eat 22 bananas in an entire day... I guess you're right - everyone is different - it is POSSIBLE to get amazing results on this diet- but not everyone is smart + capable enough to pull it off. [4]

---

4   What I find strange about the quote above is that the raw foodist seems to find it normal to have to eat 4500 calories from fruit in order to sustain this diet.

Under normal circumstances, this amount of calories is only necessary for the very top athletes. The most I can personally eat is around 3200 calories and that's only when I do some serious exercise, like training for a marathon.

It's like if someone promoted the benefits of a certain type of exercise, but in order to get the benefits, you would have to exercise for 3 hours a day instead of one. Yet, he would keep on arguing that the exercise is great and that it can give you the benefits if you're willing to give it a try and really do the work. At what point can someone say, it's not worth it?

The fact that it's extremely difficult to consume enough volume to get the calories you need on a low-fat 100% raw food diet is both an advantage and a disadvantage.

The advantage is that weight loss will be easy on this program. It's just too difficult to eat enough food!

The disadvantage is that eating this much food requires a new level of dedication, and also a capacious wallet (fruits and vegetables are not cheap).

However, if someone is dedicated enough, they will eventually train their body to eat the required quantities of fruits and vegetables to maintain their energy levels and body weight. The diet will sustain them, and it will work. And there's no denying that there are real benefits from eating this way.

But let's get back to the original topic. Eating the quantities of fruits and vegetables required to follow this lifestyle 100% requires dedication. But it will also lead to some important physiological changes.

The body will eventually get used to larger volumes of food and fiber. The stomach will stretch. Finally, the mind will adapt, and it will seem normal to eat a salad the size of a beer cooler, or drink 15 bananas in a smoothie.

When someone eats a diet like that, it's very difficult to go back and forth between raw foods and cooked foods. Like for Steve Pavlina after just a month of eating raw, small quantities of food no longer seem satisfying. Therefore, most people binge on huge quantities of cooked foods and can't understand why they can't control themselves. This is partly explained by the fact that their bodies have now adapted to a diet low in caloric density, and are now confronted with richer foods that are more easily digestible.

Physiological adaptation, and sensitivity

- **Low-salt Diet** – The body adapts to salt consumption, and it takes a few weeks to do so. Anyone who has gone on a salt-free diet can certainly attest to that. However, because of the physiological adaptations that occur on a salt-free diet, it's extremely difficult to go back and forth between a diet that contains *no* added salt and occasional consumption of foods that contain salt (like everything available in every restaurant in the world). The body needs time to adapt to salt intake, just as it needs time to adapt to a salt-free diet.

- **Digestive Enzymes** — The human body is extremely malleable. It reacts to a variety of forces and influences and to their degree of intensity. Eating certain foods makes the body produce certain digestive enzymes to digest those exact foods. That is why someone who goes vegetarian for a long period of time may find it difficult to digest meat if they choose to suddenly reintroduce it. On a raw food diet, especially one that focuses on fruit, very little digestive effort is required because fruits contain mostly simple sugars with almost no protein, and no starch or fat that require more extensive digestion. The body will slowly respond to this style of eating by "dumbing down" its digestive powers. "When you don't use it, you lose it" also applies to digesting complex meals. That is why raw foodists who go back and forth between raw and cooked find they can't digest meals that they had managed to digest perfectly just a few months before!

Reasons why a weak digestion may not be appropriate

Let's be perfectly realistic. There are times you will need to cook, or eat cooked food. In my experience, for every 100 people that have the intention of switching to a raw food diet at some point in their life and give it a good effort, less than 5 will continue eating this way for many years. And even fewer will maintain the diet 100% without exception for years on end.

So let me repeat: there are times you will need to cook, or eat cooked food. It could be every day, or every meal, or only occasionally, depending on how you decide to organize your diet and your life.

Even the strictest raw foodists that I know sometimes have to eat cooked food. It could be that they are traveling and options are limited. It could also be that they're just unable to realistically maintain a 100% raw food diet.

Achieving balance in your diet and your health should not be an all-or-nothing proposition, as many gurus would like you to believe. You should be able to occasionally make some exception to your normal program without throwing yourself completely off balance and sending your body into a feverish state of shock.

Being *that* sensitive is not a good thing.

Let's say you're traveling. One of the greatest joys of traveling abroad is experiencing new cultures. And a huge part of culture is the food people eat. I find it completely unsatisfying to travel all the way to a foreign land and not get to experience some of the food there.

Additionally, when traveling, options are generally limited. You may not find the exact same foods you find at home, so maintaining any kind of strict diet (raw foods, vegan, etc.) is a challenge. Having the possibility of making an exception once in a while is part of a normal and healthy life balance. Of course, everybody has a line they won't cross. I won't eat fried insects, or get drunk on vodka with Russian locals in a shady bar in Siberia (although I could *consider* doing both…). Some people are truly allergic to certain foods (gluten, for example). But for most of us, food choice is just a preference. And being able to make an exception to your normal preference once in a while is a healthy thing.

If you have to make an exception, your body should have enough digestive power to handle it. If you weaken your digestion so much by eating foods that require almost no digestion (like with a diet composed almost exclusively of fruits), then any meal other than what you're normally used to eating will make you sick.

I had a friend once who was a naturopath working in Montreal, who was seeing a lot of ex-raw foodists with similar problems. He told me once, "Anyone should be able to digest a meal composed of a variety of foods—carbohydrates, protein, fats."

Some raw foodists have taken the concept of purity to such an extreme that they're making their bodies constantly more sensitive and their digestion extremely delicate. They start off as raw foodists, but then refine their program by eliminating all complicated recipes and eating only fruits, vegetables, nuts and seeds. Then they eat less than 10% fat. But as their digestion weakens, they find that they feel even better when they only consume fats from avocados, and they start avoiding nuts. At some point, they feel that even the avocado is bringing their energy levels down, so they eliminate that too, achieving the diet many refer to as 90-5-5 (90% of calories from carbs, 5% from fat, 5% from protein). In this program, the only fat you're getting (less than 5%) would be contained in fruits and vegetables, all of which contain negligible amounts of fat.

Of course, with each refinement in their diet they feel better, and upon reintroducing newly forbidden foods (like nuts), they feel a "drop in energy." Essentially, they're dumbing down their digestion to the point that they can only consume foods that pass right through the system with minimal transformation. There's no doubt that such a program can increase energy levels, since so little energy is now used to digest food. However, it's a slippery slope, and this program cannot fulfill nutritional needs in the long term.

Such a person would probably feel like they'd been run over by a bus if they ate something as simple and inoffensive as a tiny bowl of cooked brown rice.

At some point, you feel like the buffet of life has been shrunk to a small table, when all you can eat is truckloads of fruit, and your body can't handle any other food. It means you can't eat out with friends for the most part. You probably can't travel, or only to places that will cater to your needs. And you create a life that is centered around food, since your main worry during the day will be how to meet your caloric needs by eating enough of those fruits and vegetables.

Putting the health and nutritional concerns of such a program aside for a while, it's quite obvious that strict raw food diets are not for everybody.

Most people will find times when they need to cook or eat cooked food. Perhaps every day, perhaps twice a day or twice a week, or just once in a while. But it will happen. Therefore, it's important to design a diet that allows you a little flexibility, and also one that allows your digestion to be strong enough to handle what comes your way.

Avoiding Fear and Scarcity Around Food

When I was a strict raw foodist, I lived in a state of fear. I had to worry about my raw food meals, but I also had to worry about what might happen if I ate something cooked.

I am a very passionate person and I have many interests in life. I could be described as a "Renaissance man." I have intense involvement in music, language, business, writing, food, nutrition, and many other things.

Some people are perfectionists. Once they find something to be passionate about, they stick to it and it becomes their life. They learn to play a musical instrument, and then make a career out of it, and music becomes their life.

Or they discover the raw food diet, find out how to do it 100%, and never look back.

I am not such a person. I could never say that I'm going to do something 100% for the rest of my life, or completely give up something that I used to love without ever looking back.

When I was a raw foodist, making an exception was not fun. First, I couldn't control myself, and would often "binge" and eat way more than what my body needed. But even if I managed to control myself, I generally felt at least guilty if not sick from my indulgence.

Now there are still things that I don't generally eat, but I haven't crossed any food completely off the list. For example, I generally don't eat chocolate. I find chocolate too stimulating and I'm just not fond of it in general. But occasionally I might have a piece of chocolate. If a friend just came back from a trip to Switzerland bringing me the gift of perfect chocolate that I absolutely have to try, then I will eat some.

I generally don't eat fried food. It's unhealthy, for one thing, and I don't like grease. For example, French fries are something I generally don't eat. I don't make them, I don't go out of my way to eat them, and I don't crave them. But there could be an occasion when I might eat a few French fries. Maybe I'm in Belgium, and I'm with a friend who's in the mood for French fries.

Another food I generally don't consume is milk. Although in the case of dairy, I'm actually very fond of yogurt, especially Greek yogurt, so it's not something that leaves me completely indifferent. However, I'm aware of the problems with overconsumption of dairy products, and I feel at my best when I don't have them. But this doesn't mean that dairy is completely out of the question on special occasions. I'm not lactose intolerant, and nothing majorly wrong will happen to me if I have a bit of yogurt one day or bit of milk in some coffee. I'm also not in the habit of eating ice cream. I almost never eat it, I never purchase it (not even the natural or vegan versions), but once in a while, I will eat a scoop of ice cream.

The Two Rules That Have Liberated My Life

I have two basic rules that have literally lifted a HUGE burden off my shoulders and made my life much more fun, removed a huge amount of stress and, honestly, have only been positive. The rules are:

If I'm invited to eat somewhere, I don't make a special request. I eat whatever is offered to me, and I'm grateful for it.

When I'm on vacation, I eat whatever I feel like eating.

Let me put the rules in perspective so you understand. If I were frequently invited for dinner, maybe my rule would be different. But because these invitations are generally limited to two-to-three times a month, I'm very happy with my relaxed approach. All the stress and discomfort of explaining dietary restrictions to my hosts is removed, and I actually enjoy my time a lot more. So far, none of my hosts has tried to poison me, and I've always felt great after those dinners. If things changed and most of my hosts made dishes filled with melted cheese, then maybe I'd change the rule. But so far, the rule has worked out for me because foods served by my hosts and friends has generally been healthy; certainly something I could eat once or twice a month without affecting my health in any negative way.

As for vacations, my rule applies to times when I travel purely for pleasure. I don't apply the rule to business trips. I tend to travel a lot, but only once or twice a year will I take a "true vacation." And my rule allows me to completely relax and enjoy myself during that time. The rule is simple: I'll eat whatever I feel like eating. It doesn't mean I HAVE to eat all the junk food I can find. If I feel like eating fruits and veggies, I'll eat fruits and veggies. If I feel like having pizza in Italy at the hole-in-the-wall restaurant all the locals are raving about, then I'll have pizza there.

Why have the rules

If, like me, you come from a background of obsession with diet — maybe you've seriously experimented with veganism or raw foodism, the "rules" will seem outrageous to you.

I can already hear the objections:

"How could you eat pizza? It's so bad for you!"

"I can't believe that Frederic Patenaude admits to eating ice cream!"

"Moderation in all things is a philosophy that's making people sick!"

"I could never eat dead animals!"

I know, I know. I understand all the objections, and I've been through it all. For a raw foodist, diet is the be-all and end-all of all health pursuits. And in order to achieve paradise health or whatever the next level is thought to be, certain things have to be black and white. Either you're a "carnivore" or you're a "vegan." You're either "raw" or "cooked." It's all or nothing, and you're supposed to only move upward with diet, not take backward steps like I'm doing with such a liberal set of rules.

But here's where the rules can help you. For a very small minority of people, sticking to a diet 100% without making any exception is easy. Doing it even makes these people happy.

For another group of people, sticking to a diet is a matter of life and death. These people could have a life-threatening disease and need to follow a certain set of guidelines without ever making any exception.

My "rules" are not meant for these people. Rather, they have worked for me, and I know they will work for a large group of people who feel that the philosophy of "100%" in diet is just suffocating them—whether they realize they're feeling this way or not!

I can only share my own experience.

For years, I would follow a mostly raw, plant-based diet and occasionally would make an exception or, as some people would say, "cheated" on my diet.

Now, I still follow a mostly raw, plant-based diet, and also eat on occasion a few things I wouldn't normally eat. The only difference is that I've removed all the guilt and struggle associated with these exceptions. I lifted a huge burden off my shoulders when I decided that I could be invited somewhere and make absolutely no special request about what was served. I could stop being a pain in the ass! And I could also travel with very few dietary restrictions and just enjoy myself.

Believe me: you still get to make choices. When I travel, I don't randomly eat every bit of junk food that comes my way. Instead, I eat *what I feel like eating*. Because I follow certain principles that keep me healthy, as I will discuss in other parts of this book, a few indulgences are not going to make a big difference to the big picture. I want to make choices that are going to *add* to my quality of life, not detract from it. And part of what defines good quality of life for me is the ability to experience new things when I'm traveling, and to have freedom to breathe when I'm invited to dinner or eat out with friends at a restaurant.

If I'm in Italy, I'm going to have some gelato. And in In Italy, the gelato serving size is about a third the size of that sold in America. Yes, gelato contains dairy (a rather small amount, indeed), and dairy is something that I *generally* avoid. But when in Rome, I do a little bit like the Romans, and I will have some gelato.

This is not the modern idea of "moderation"

My little rules are not really like the modern concept of "everything in moderation." I admit that the concept of moderation has been adulterated and used as an excuse by most people in the West, to the point that it no longer means anything.

People like to say that they want to "enjoy everything in moderation" when in fact what they mean is "I want to eat whatever the heck I want."

Most Americans, despite what they say, are not enjoying the good things of life "in moderation." And the proof is in the pudding. If you look at the results, most people still have quite a long way to go before they can claim they are actually moderate people.

Raw foodists, on the other hand, tend to be extreme people. They see things as black and white, as "healthy" or "disease-causing."

What I've realized over time is that certain things are making people sick because of how frequently they are eaten. For example, when I first became a raw foodist, I would eat massive quantities of avocados, nuts and seeds. This actually made me sick. Now does that mean that nuts and seeds and avocados are unhealthy? Of course not. But when I first became a raw foodist, I would sometimes eat several avocados a day. Nowadays, I couldn't imagine eating more than half an avocado at any one time.

I knew raw foodists that would polish off half a jar of almond butter in a single day. This is more than too much for that category of food.

And because raw foodists have forgotten how to properly balance their diet, they want to see everything as black and white. There are certain foods they can *never* eat, but they're grossly overeating other foods.

If you're reading this book, it means you're probably not interested in following a 100% raw food diet for the rest of your life. You're looking for something in between pure raw foodism and a "healthy diet." If not, then I would say you're reading the wrong book!

Part of designing a healthy diet is learning to be moderate, in the *true* sense of the word. This means having a balanced lifestyle with some diet guidelines that work for you, but with some breathing room to make occasional exceptions.

Why no restriction like "vegan" etc.

Some people might wonder why they couldn't just eat a plant-based diet that includes a lot of raw foods, and perhaps allow themselves to eat richer cooked foods on occasion but still stay vegan.

I can only talk about my own experience. Nowhere am I suggesting that you stop being a vegetarian if that's important to you, or that you follow my rules if they don't work for you. You have to create your *own* set of rules that are adapted to your *own* life circumstances.

My circumstances are that I'm a 37-year old guy who became a vegetarian at the age of 18, then went raw, and maintained a never-ending passion/obsession with diet and nutrition ever since. Although I did not remain a pure vegetarian for all these years, or a pure raw foodist for that matter, and had many phases of experimentation, I always reverted to either veganism or pure raw foodism, or something in between.

I've never had any issues with my weight, except in my early days as a raw foodist when I was actually underweight.

I also love traveling and discovering foreign cultures; and building a good social life and relationship with my family is something that's important to me.

When I'm traveling, I walk at least 8 miles a day, on average. So eating *whatever I feel like* actually works in that context.

I also don't have any *real* allergy to any food.

So again, my rules work for me.

Whenever I'm invited out for dinner, at a friend's house for example, I eat whatever is on the menu and I don't make any special requests.

When I'm traveling for pleasure, I eat whatever I feel like eating.

These two rules truly WORK for me. They've totally liberated my life. And I can say that the overall quality of my life has truly improved since I've been following these rules.

The rules have also taught me the value of *true* moderation. When I was going back and forth between a pure raw food diet and eating cooked food, I would feel horrible every time I "cheated." Not only did my body violently react to these foods, but I would also grossly overeat. I could not restrict myself to one little taste of something. But now, moderation is easy. That's because my body has adjusted to being able to digest a wider variety of foods, and my mind no longer feels the lack of certain foods, so I'm not as tempted to overeat.

It's important that you find some rules that liberate you. They have to work in the context of your *own* life and circumstances. Maybe my rules will work for you, maybe they won't, but you should establish some guidelines that both liberate you and keep you healthy.

Consistency is Key

There is one important concept I'd like you to get out of this book as you experience the following benefits:

- Great health and immunity
- Excellent digestion
- Great energy
- An ideal weight and the ability to maintain it
- Emotional balance and stability

This key is *consistency*. It's very important to get out of the "YO-YO" mentality — always going back and forth between extremes.

An example of the "yo-yo" lifestyle would be to eat 100% raw or pretty close to it, but cheat on the weekends and feel bad about it (and feel physically terrible). Or always try to go on new cleanses, detox programs, and fasts.

You need to find balance. You need to develop a consistent routine and stick to it.

This is why what some people call the 95% raw food diet doesn't work. It's better to either stick to a 100% raw food diet — all the time — and in fact stick to a *consistent* raw food diet, than to go back and forth constantly.

For most people, as we've seen, a 100% raw food diet is not appropriate. So what we need to do is to design a plan that incorporates the level of raw foods that you feel comfortable with, as well as the right balance of nutrients, and then stick to it. Eat some cooked food every day. Don't just occasionally binge at restaurants. Stay consistent, and your digestion will improve, your moods will get better, and you will experience stability.

How to Keep the Digestive Juices Flowing

There are a few things you can eat that will help build your digestive power so that you are not so sensitive anytime you eat something outside of your "normal ideal guidelines."

Unfortunately, very little scientific research exists on this topic since interest in extreme diets among the scientific community is almost non-existent. Very few people actually follow a 100% raw food diet for decades, and almost no studies have been done on the long-term effects of this diet.

So the following observations are based on my personal experience and that of other raw foodists I have met and interviewed over the years.

If you've been following a very restricted diet for an extensive period of time, it's likely that your body has temporarily lost some digestive "memory" and needs to be patiently retrained in order to operate properly again.

The level of retraining will depend on the level of restriction you've imposed on yourself, and for how long you've done it. In my first few years as a raw foodist, I did not restrict fat (such as nuts), but I did restrict all condiments. That is why simply going to a raw food restaurant where condiments were used would "make me feel like crap."

There are essentially a few categories of food — whole macronutrient classes, in fact — that need to be reintroduced carefully in order for digestive juices to flow normally again. They are:

Salt — This one has nothing to do with digestion, but more with how the body regulates sodium intake. Although going salt-free has its benefits, using a little bit of salt on your food will make you able to at least withstand eating out, where salt is used massively.

Protein — This category includes all animal protein, but also concentrated sources of vegetable protein, such as tofu. The inability to digest protein will be noticed when these foods are expelled from the body almost undigested and with an unusual amount of bile in the stools.

Fat — If you've eliminated all fats for a while (nuts, oils, avocados, etc.) your body will need some retraining in order to be able to digest those foods again. You can tell your body has lost its ability to digest fats when you feel like you're about to die after eating a fatty meal.

Cooked starches — The body can also get weakened in ability to digest cooked starches. This manifests itself in unusual tiredness and sleepiness after even a small amount of starch (for example, a cup of rice).

Readjusting to Salt

A very basic thing that can be done to prevent much of the "feel like shit" feelings when cheating on a rather pure diet is consuming *some* salt on a regular basis. The body is expert at adapting to sodium intake. But if it changes dramatically, you can be in trouble.

I do believe that a relatively low-sodium diet can be very healthy, but it's not very practical in the real world. Lots of foods are simply not that enjoyable to eat without a little salt, and you're bound to come across added salt in almost any meal eating out.

How much sodium is healthy? Previous recommendations put the upper limit at 2300 mg. a day for most people. Now the ideal limit is 1500 mg. a day. There are, of course, passionate debates within the alternative health community on this very topic.

But even if you wanted to stick to official recommendations, your food already contains 500 mg. of sodium (naturally occurring in fruits, vegetables, grains and other foods), which means you could add an extra 1000 mg. of sodium a day. That's a little less than half a teaspoon of salt per day. That's a small amount, but generous enough to not feel completely deprived and enjoy a little salty kick to your food.

I personally consume more sodium than this, because I don't pay that much attention to it anymore. The reason is that at this point, I want to enjoy food and not obsess about it so much. My breakfast is almost always a green smoothie, and sometimes oatmeal; two meals that don't contain any extra salt. I almost always prepare foods I eat myself, and I control the amount of salt that I eat. However, I don't restrict myself with it.

Protein

A few years ago, I met a very enthusiastic raw foodist who followed some principles of instinctive nutrition. He ate a diet composed exclusively of raw foods, but very occasionally ate some animal foods.

His observation was that his occasional consumption of protein in the form of animal foods strengthened his digestion. Even if it was occasional, he noticed that after eating some animal foods, his digestion was more powerful and efficient afterwards, in the days or weeks following his small protein meals.

This could be because protein foods stimulate hydrochloric acid production. A low-fat raw food diet is a very low-protein diet; therefore one that stimulates very little production of digestive enzymes and hydrochloric acid. When a raw foodist goes off the wagon with a cooked meal, she's rarely able to digest it properly because her system is no longer used to digesting more complex substances.

I've also noticed that consumption of protein foods strengthens digestion. For many years, my digestion was absolutely horrible on a mostly raw food diet (low in fat, high in fruit). In other respects my results were great, but my stools were very loose, almost watery most of the time. I would get an urgent need to go to the bathroom after many meals.

Then I changed my eating plan, and stopped eating large quantities of fruit for a while as an experiment. I also consumed protein foods in the form of beans, rather small quantities of tofu, and some animal foods (mainly some fish, and some meat).

After that experiment, I went back to try a 100% raw food diet composed almost exclusively of fruit, with some salads. In the past, eating this way would have caused very watery, urgent stools. But after my experiment eliminating most of my fruit intake and consuming protein foods for a while, I experienced wonderful digestion eating a fruit-based diet.

I ate huge quantities of fruit, and my digestion was perfect. I did not experience any of the symptoms that bothered me in the past.

My conclusion is that it's possible to strengthen digestive power, as long as it's not always dumbed down by an overly simple diet. Protein-rich foods consumed once a day or on occasion will strengthen digestion. If your goal is to be able to digest a wider variety of foods, you should consider adding some protein foods. The amounts need not be very large, and for animal foods, it's not necessary to consume them every day.

Keep in mind that some foods, such as nuts and seeds, are considered "protein foods" but are actually sources of fat. A protein food is a food where most of the calories come from protein. In the vegetable realm, that generally means soy products (tofu and other meat substitutes).

If you're a former raw foodist who wants to stay vegan, I would suggest adding some tofu and soy-based meat substitutes to your diet for a little while. Even if you're not planning to eat these foods in the future, it will benefit your digestion and help retrain it to handle a wider variety of foods.

It's possible, if you've been following a rather restricted diet for a while, that you won't be able to fully digest these foods at first. But your digestion will strengthen over time, just like a muscle growing bigger with use. You need to start VERY slowly. 2 ounces is a good start, but increase gradually; there's no need to consume more than 4-6 ounces of protein foods at once.

Protein needs are estimated at 0.8 grams per kilogram of body weight, or 7 grams per 20 pounds. So a male weighing 160 pounds would need 56 grams of protein a day. Athletes need closer to 1 gram per kg, or 9 g per 20 pounds. That would be 72 grams for the same person.

It's certainly possible to get this amount of protein on a raw food diet. However, caloric intake for athletic people needs to be high — in fact 15-25% higher than it would have to be on a diet that included cooked food.

Raw foodists, including myself, have often claimed that protein deficiencies are non-existent in the Western world. That's true. However other symptoms of low protein intake are possible even in the West. Inadequate protein intake is almost always paired with inadequate caloric intake. On a raw food diet, adequate caloric intake is a challenge; therefore symptoms of low protein intake are possible. While this is not a true "protein deficiency," it can lead to some health problems.

In my experience, athletes dedicated to a low-fat raw vegan diet are generally motivated to eat the quantities of fruit necessary to make this diet work, and therefore manage to get the proper amounts of calories they need. As we've seen, that's 15-25% more than on normal diets.

However, symptoms of low protein intake do occur in many people following a raw food diet, particularly children, who need more protein (and calories) for growth. For that reason, I absolutely do not recommend a raw food diet for children under any circumstances.

Symptoms of low protein intake include:
- Muscle wasting
- Unwanted weight loss
- Fatigue and weakness
- Frequent infections
- Severe edema (fluid retention)
- Slow growth and development in children

Again, I would not say that raw foodists necessarily experience symptoms of low protein intake. But many do. Increasing overall calories consumed is generally a good idea, but this cannot work for many people. Why?

- Many people are sensitive to the acids in fruits and cannot consume large quantities without experiencing severe enamel erosion.
- Fruit-based diets can also cause many dental problems in susceptible individuals, more than any other diet.
- Many people simply cannot eat the quantities necessary to sustain a raw food diet.
- Growing children and many athletes simply cannot get the amounts of protein necessary for optimal health and growth on a raw food diet.

In the context of strengthening digestion, starting small and staying consistent for a while eating at least 2-3 ounces of protein foods every day will help you make tremendous gains in strengthening your digestion.

Fats

Deficiency is usually not a problem, as most raw foodists tend to eat more of their calories from fat than any other macronutrient. However, it could be a problem for people who try to restrict their fat intake to less than 10% or even 5% of total calories.

There is a new tendency within the raw food movement to go

"90-5-5." People following this diet eat only fruits and vegetables and use no added fats of any kind. No avocados, nuts, seeds or oils.

Because fruits and vegetables seldom contain more than 5% of their calories from either fat or protein, the macronutrient breakdown of the diet is: 90-5-5.[5]

If you've followed such a program for a good period of time, or even just consume fatty foods infrequently, you will have some fat-digesting retraining to do.

---

5   90% carbohydrates, 5% fat and 5% protein.

Nut butters are probably the best place to start, as they are relatively easy to digest and contain many essential nutrients. Start with one ounce a day, and build from there, until you can easily digest 50 grams of fat a day (which would be about six tablespoons of almond butter, for example). Of course, mix it up with other fat sources, such as avocados, and even a little bit of olive oil.

Starches

Starches are some of the easiest foods for the human body to digest and assimilate. Yet, if you've been abstaining from them, you will find it challenging to eat your old comfort foods such as potatoes, rice or beans. The main symptom is a feeling of extreme tiredness after eating even a conservative amount of starch, or a sort of "hungover" feeling the next day.

The good news is that your body can easily be retrained to digest starch. Start with root vegetables, such as potatoes, and then move on to rice and beans. However, make sure you restrict yourself to a small quantity at first. You don't want to sit down to eat two or three pounds of cooked potatoes and then complain later that these foods are evil because they make you feel so tired!

Gluten

There is a trend in the natural food industry whereby everybody self-diagnoses himself or herself as "gluten-intolerant" or "gluten-sensitive." Celiac disease is no laughing matter, but although issues with gluten, and particularly wheat, are real, most people are not as gluten-intolerant as they think they are. Generally, their health has been assaulted on all fronts so that gluten is just one more thing that adds to the mix.

Unless you are truly gluten-intolerant, in which case you should abstain from wheat products and other gluten sources completely, there's a good chance that you should be able to handle a little wheat without too many problems.

If you stop eating wheat products completely, your body may give you signals that you could mistake for true gluten sensitivity. In fact, it could just be that you've temporarily lost your ability to digest those foods properly.

Don't get me wrong: modern wheat is an abomination and most people would be far better off if they ate less of it or avoided it completely. However, wheat is also part of life. There's no way you can be part of "normal life" and avoid wheat completely, without it being a complete hassle. If you're not sure about that, just ask anyone who's truly Celiac if they think avoiding wheat makes life easier.

Realistically, most people are going to want to be able to eat wheat products once in a while. So I would suggest in the initial stages of your "diet rehabilitation" that you include some wheat products. Do this after you've started retraining your body to digest every other category of food.

The key with wheat is moderation. It's best if products like bread and wheat pasta are not part of your normal, *regular* diet. But again, wheat is part of modern life. You're going to encounter it. Maybe it's going to be that bagel that your aging aunt would really be happy if you shared with her, or simply the hidden gluten that's in almost every restaurant food you're likely to come across. You just can't completely run away from gluten! So it's better to build some tolerance for it.

Removing the Guilt and the Quest for Perfection

After having immersed yourself in healthy diets and the concept of raw foodism, it's normal to see food differently and experience guilt when returning to cooked foods, especially if you've practiced strict raw foodism for a long period of time.

People who have been *trying* for years to eat a raw food diet and consider a 100% raw diet their *ideal* find it especially difficult not to think they've been a failure and lacking in discipline when it comes to this aspect of their lives.

Some readers sent me these emails:

> "I would love to be able to eat cooked food without guilt. I believe my body responds well to a totally raw diet, but after my two years was up, I was seduced by cooked. I eat both now, but worry about it."

> "I don't think it's a good idea to be fanatic trying to eat absolutely 100% raw, especially in the beginning. I don't get much pocket money, so it'd be pretty impossible for me to get all the things I need to transition to a high raw food diet at once (like a high quality blender, good raw recipe books, support forum membership and such). So I still eat cooked food every day (but also much more fruits and salad than before) and I DON'T feel guilty about it. I think that one of the most important things about eating and feeling good is to never think anything bad about what you're putting in your mouth. Thoughts like "I shouldn't be eating this burger 'cause it'll ruin my health, but oh well I can't help myself" or "Yuck, this broccoli tastes awful but I've just got to eat it 'cause it's healthy" will actually make the food worse. I've decided that if I can't enjoy eating something, I won't eat it at all. But luckily I like the taste of most raw fruits and veggies."

It's very easy to think that the only reason you haven't been successful with a 100% raw food diet is just because *you haven't tried hard enough.* This opinion is often reinforced by those promoting their own agenda and opinions, as well as the few people that consider themselves successful with this lifestyle.

And in some cases, it's possible that people have not given the diet a fair try. But in most cases, I would say they're trying to hold on to a lifestyle that simply does not work for them, and certainly isn't making them happy.

To illustrate my point, here's a quote from one of the numerous posts from raw foodists asking others for help on raw food forums:

"Hi Everyone, I have been trying to do the raw food lifestyle since April with some success and health benefits but I am having trouble going all the way. Eating 100% raw all the time and basing my diet on fruit seems out of my reach. I get horrible cooked foods cravings and sometimes feel that I can't control myself. Today I binged and ate the worst foods and was rewarded with horrible cramping and diarrhea. I feel very discouraged and wonder if this is not for me :(I have trouble staying motivated and excited for fruit. I want the benefits of this lifestyle but what do I need to do to stay in control and look forward to lots of fresh fruit. Some days I get very bored and I don't want to eat at all. Any tips would be appreciated."

Here are some of the replies she got:

- "Undereat and you will binge. Eat enough fruit and you'll be satisfied."
- "Sometimes you might have to pretend that fruit and veg are the only choices available."
- "This diet only gets easier the more you practice it."
- "You should consider coming to my raw food retreat so you can meet likeminded people."
- "It does take a lot of practice. Just don't give up!"
- "You're probably undereating, just track your calories using an online application."

The person who posted asking for health advice said things I think are quite representative of how many people feel in this movement. One thing she asked about that wasn't answered by any of the advice she got on the forum was her actual discouragement and boredom, and lack of desire to eat. In other words, eating this way was not making her happy, and she wasn't looking forward to the same repetitive meals. At the same time, she was suffering from that fact that the diet requires extraordinary commitment (such as having to travel far away to meet likeminded people, tracking calories, and learning to eat huge volumes of food in order to be content and avoid cravings; and not being able to *ever* cheat on the diet without being rewarded with horrible cramps and diarrhea.

The issue of her body reacting so negatively after a cooked meal is something that none of the comments she got in response addressed properly. She also mentioned that eating this diet seemed "out of her reach," yet everybody tried to convince her that she simply wasn't trying hard enough.

It's true that one of the main challenges of a raw food diet, especially a fruit based one, is getting enough calories. When consuming enough calories, it's possible to avoid cravings for cooked foods.

However, this doesn't change the fact that making this diet work requires extraordinary commitment, and when the rewards are not clear, one must question whether it is actually worth it to try such an austere lifestyle.

Stress

Sometimes, you can find happiness if you let go of dogma. One reader sent me the following insightful email:

> I'm generally against as you call it "fanaticism", but I do consider healthy eating as much as comfortably possible to be a must. I come from a Mediterranean climate and I eat sea food, olive oil, eggs, pasta etc., but mostly I try to eat salads, green smoothies, vegetables, fruits, legumes, sprouts, grains etc. I do consume milk but we have our own goats, so I don't use store-bought dairy. I like your articles and I choose to follow what I can and what I consider to be rational and good for me. I think there's one more side to

consider in all this food obsession, and that is stress. If choice of food makes you stressful then all the benefits are almost gone, swallowed by stress. So do some active living, breathing, do some meditation; doesn't need to be yoga, can be "thought-less" walks in the woods or by the sea, and always take the healthier choice between two foods and you'll be good to go. I chose to live like this a couple of years ago and I've never been more healthy, happy, holy and relaxed. Life always finds a way to get to you, at least a little bit, but this is as good as it gets, for me! Hope I offered a little insight of my own.

How to Break Free from the Prison Called "The Raw Food Diet"

People who eat a 100% raw food diet and have done it for years and are happy about it live in a world of their own. They've learned what it takes to be successful with the diet, they are happy about the benefits they are getting, and they feel that the sacrifices they had to make were worth it for them.

It could be that some people simply have the type of personality that makes it easier for them to stick to one thing and never look back. Other people, like me, have a curious nature, are always interested in new things, and simply can't conceive of living life in such a rigid and regimented way. For such people, a 100% raw food diet is a prison that they can't break free from. They may eventually get to like their diet, but for whatever reason, they often feel tempted to eat other things. Every little exception is rewarded with extreme feelings of sickness, cramps, bad digestion, and the general feeling that the Gods of Raw Foods are really unhappy about their cheating and are massively punishing them. At the same time, everyone who's supposedly following a 100% raw food diet tells them that the only reason they are not happy with the diet or not successful with it is because they haven't tried enough. Yet, people who are struggling feel they have already made extraordinary efforts but, as the poster on the forum said, it just seems "beyond my reach."

Nothing is wrong with you if you decide that a 100% raw food diet is beyond your reach. In fact, it is not realistically an appropriate diet for 99% of people. What matters is that if you make certain sacrifices, you are rewarded in proportion to the level of sacrifice you make. In other words, you need to calculate the return on investment of a raw food diet.

Calculating the ROI of a raw food diet

In business, calculating the ROI (return on investment) of an expense is a very important part of the process. A company can't just spend millions of dollars on advertising. It needs to know that whatever money it is investing will have an adequate ROI. Millions spent on advertising should result in even more millions in sales. Otherwise, the money is wasted and the company will go under. Each expense, such as the salary paid to employees, the advertising budget, the training of employees, must be examined and the ROI established. That's why companies will sometimes spend tens of millions of dollars on the salary of a new CEO. Although most people outside the company see this as a non-egalitarian measure, in most cases, CEOs being paid that much money have the skills to turn the company around and bring in so much more than what they are being paid in salary. So, unfair as it seems, a highly paid, highly competent CEO brings a much better ROI for a company than any other business expense.

You're not a company. But you can still examine the ROI of certain personal "investments" in your own life.

For example, you decide to get in shape, and work out four or five times a week at the gym, or outside. You'll have to give up four or five hours of your life every week, and will experience some initial discomfort. But like most people, you'll probably find that these four or five hours are an investment that provides a very good "return" because you're getting better health, a more beautiful body, better sleep, and more.

You can also calculate the ROI of your diet. What are you getting "in return" for what you're giving up?

Most raw food gurus and their committed followers want you to believe that a 100% raw food diet is almost a *no-brainer*. It is *so* much better for you that you would be a fool not to do it. In fact, it is expected that you expend extraordinary efforts to do it, and do it well, under all circumstances, because the benefits are so awesome and extraordinary.

The main question to ask yourself is whether the benefits that you get from a 100% raw food diet are so worth it to you — and couldn't possibly come from any other diet that would be less restrictive — and worth all the sacrifices you are making. Is there a positive ROI?

Some people may very well answer *yes* to that question. But maybe this answer will change at some point in the future.

When I asked myself the question, I realized that a 100% raw food diet was simply not appropriate for me.

My ROI table looked like this…

What I'm Giving Up:

- I have to give up eating a wide variety of foods, many of which I love.
- I have to give up a lot of the pleasure of eating.
- I'm not actually happy eating a 100% raw food diet. I find it too restrictive.
- I feel cold during the winter, and cannot comfort myself by eating something warm.
- I cannot have an easy social life.
- My dental health is going down. My teeth are more sensitive and prone to cavities.
- I cannot eat at restaurants, unless I jump through major hoops, which makes it an unpleasant experience.
- I cannot enjoy a fun night of food and wine with friends.

- I am limited to dating people compatible with my diet philosophy, which is a very small pool of people.
- I have to constantly think about food to ensure I don't run out. There's much more planning involved to make the diet successful.
- I have to eat massive quantities of food.
- The diet costs me a lot more money.
- My digestion is not optimal.
- I cannot "cheat" without feeling like crap.

What I'm Getting in Return

- I have good energy and find it easier to exercise than with my previous diet.
- There's a good chance I will avoid many degenerative diseases, due to the fact that I don't consume the foods that are making most people sick.

So as you can see, my list of benefits was very slim, but my list of negatives was long indeed.

The next thing I asked myself is, "Could I possibly get these benefits from a less restrictive diet?" I also asked myself whether the benefits I was experiencing came from the fact that I was *not* eating certain foods or whether it was actually *because* I was eating a 100% raw food diet.

What I determined was that I could actually get all the same benefits and none of the negatives with a less restrictive diet.

And what I will show you in this book is that science does not actually support many of the arguments used by raw foodists to promote their lifestyle. A diet that incorporates plenty of raw foods, fruits and vegetables, AND avoids for the most part the foods that are making most people sick, is conducive to great health, great fitness performance, and most of the benefits people are seeking from a raw food diet.

I am not a top athlete. Therefore, I cannot tell you whether I am performing at my best on my current diet or if I could perform better on a 100% raw food diet. But the truth is, this does not matter to me. For my level of activity — working out five or six times a week — my current diet provides me just as much energy as a 100% raw food diet. In fact, I find that I make progress with weight training much faster now than I ever did on a 100% raw diet.

It is important to determine the ROI of a raw food diet, or any other restricted diet. Are you getting the results you desire? *Can* you get the results you desire? And most important, are you okay with what you're giving up in order to get these results, and could these results be obtained without giving up those things?

Cleansing vs. Maintenance Diets

"The more rules you set for people's eating, and the more you rage against some kind of tyranny (real or perceived: think wheat, sugar, or, in the recent past, saturated fats), the more people take up your flag and wave it alongside you."

Cleanses are all the rage, in all forms of the raw food diet — fruitarian, low-fat, living foods, etc.

We can see it when we look at all the efforts that people following these diets are making to get past the state loosely called "detox" to the hallowed place of complete purity, although many who strive for this also come to believe that the world is so toxic and themselves so imperfect that the detox must be never-ending.

Whether it's juice "feasting," water fasting, fasting once a week, green juices, the elimination of all fats, food combining, or other disciplines, there seems to be no end to the attempts to continually cleanse the body.

This stems from a belief that the human body is fundamentally a machine that should run very clean. Under appropriate circumstances, the human body would never experience any gas, have any unpleasant body odor, or feel "congested" or "clogged up" in any way.

There is also the belief that years of unhealthy eating habits somehow do the same damage to the body as putting the wrong kind of oil in a car. Over time, things get clogged up, so it's necessary to clean things up every so often.

Although there are some flaws in this reasoning — we'll talk about them in just a moment — there's nothing wrong with wanting to give your body or digestion a rest once in a while. Just a little fasting or some sort of "detox" diet as part of your overall health plan can be beneficial, although what actually happens when someone goes on a detox diet is very far from the sort of "cellular cleansing" benefits that are claimed.

The human body is not like a machine that can be cleaned up from the inside using special products. The green juices you put in your body are not literally "cleaning you out." They're used as nutrition just like any other food. Your own cells continually produce waste materials every hour of the day, and the body works at removing them non-stop. What you eat doesn't affect this process that much, but giving your body a digestive rest may well give it extra energy to help in the healing process, in many cases.

Using some periodic fasting as part of your health routine is something that is actually proven to extend life — more than any other practice that has been studied by scientists. "Fasting" can be understood as a form of caloric restriction. A juice fast or green smoothie diet, although not as extreme as a water fast — are also forms of caloric restriction. And it is primarily this caloric restriction that does the job of helping the body live longer and more disease-free.

Problems arise when you take these forms of fasting or "cleansing" and turn them into a full-time lifestyle. And that is also the main reason why many raw foodists experience health decline after many years on the diet. They've taken their obsession for detox diets too far and forgotten that the body also needs maintenance and balance.

The Obsession with Purity

A characteristic of people on raw food diets is this constant obsession with purity. It's something that's been oversold by raw food gurus when they described the promised benefits of following this lifestyle.

Not only will you lose weight and have more energy, they say, but you will also:

- Eliminate any body odor — raw foodists don't need to use deodorant!
- Have pleasant-smelling stools, almost like roses coming out of a garden!

- Never even need to use toilet paper!
- Never experience unpleasant gas or other symptoms of indigestion.
- Have breath that smells like fruit.

Because raw foodists actually expect all these things to happen as a matter of course, they think something is wrong when they pass a little gas or have a bit of body odor after eating nuts.

So then they resolve to be even stricter. They eliminate nuts from their diet and get even stricter with food combining, while stepping up their already aggressive herbal or colonic cleansing protocols.

But is the human body truly supposed to run that clean?

A person who has taken their "purity" to its logical conclusion will be able to digest only very few things, in only very specific combinations. He might sigh, "I'm so sensitive," like a martyr to the goal of inner cleanliness. The truth is, there's a difference between sensitivity and *reactivity*. This person is not sensitive, but reactive. Sensitivity is a very flexible way of being, whereby the body senses the conditions at hand and adapts to them. Reactivity is not at all flexible, and whereas sensitivity is a strength, reactivity is a disadvantage.

As I was breaking free of some of my negative brainwashing as a raw foodist, I found it very important to understand that I did not need to seek absolute bodily purity in the sense many raw foodists understand it.

Although I do find that my digestion is overall a lot better on my current diet than when I was following a 100% raw food diet, there are times when I need to use a deodorant, but this doesn't mean that my body is the pit of eternal stench.

Cleansing vs. Maintenance Diets

Certain diets are appropriate for short-term, cleansing purposes. Just like you wouldn't fast or drink only juices for the rest of your life, you wouldn't follow a diet that is too light and simple for the rest of your life, because this is not a good maintenance diet. A diet of fruits and vegetables with absolutely no fats (no avocados, nuts or seeds at all) may well work as a nice detox diet or almost a limited form of fasting, but it's not an appropriate diet to maintain and build the human body over long period of times. The proof is that growing children and pregnant women, who need higher levels of nutrition to fuel growth, are not advised to eat this type of diet.

Sometimes your body needs something lighter. Sometimes you need to give your digestion a break. But to build health, you also need to provide your body some solid, easily digestible nutrition most of the time. A diet of sprouts, salads and a little fruit sounds great and rejuvenating on paper, but it's not something that can sustain human beings across all phases of their lives.

The best way to monitor whether the diet you've been eating is a little too close to a cleansing diet rather than a proper maintenance diet is to observe your cravings. Unless you follow an extremely unhealthy diet or are a recovering addict of some kind, cravings are generally an indication that your body is *lacking* something. The stronger your cravings, the more likely that that "*something*" is just *calories*.

We've already seen that raw fruits and vegetables yield fewer useable calories than similar cooked foods, and the difference can be as much as 20 or 25%. On top of that, fruits and vegetables have a low caloric density, making it hard to meet your energy needs unless you're making astounding efforts to pack in the calories, by eating things like a 15-banana smoothie or lots of dried fruit, which can be hard on the teeth and can cause diarrhea, which is counterproductive. This is one of the main reasons children should never eat a raw food diet, especially not a strict one that avoids all fats. Their energy needs are too high and their stomachs too small to handle the necessary volume to thrive on a raw food diet.

The question I'll inevitably get asked is "If you can get enough calories, isn't a diet of fruits and vegetables okay?"

I think asking the question is answering it already. It's almost like saying "I know it's extremely difficult, but let's imagine that by some extraordinary effort I succeeded in getting all the calories I needed from just fruits and vegetables, would that be okay?"

The answer is "Maybe." Some people certainly thrive on such a program, but it remains to be seen how long their good health can last. The reported rate of failure on this kind of diet is very high, which means it's not as easy as it sounds.

The problem comes when the people who claim to be in the handful that actually thrive on fat-free raw food diets think of themselves as some sort of elite, and look down on people not able to follow their program. "You're just not trying hard enough," they seem to say to people who claim to have failed on their program. "I told you to get 3500 calories from fruits and vegetables every day. You didn't do it. That's not because my program doesn't work. It's because you didn't make the diet work!"

Some people will also say "But Fred, didn't *you* always recommend a low-fat diet based on fruits and vegetables?"

To which I will respond, "There's a difference between "low-fat" and "fat-free."

I *never* recommended the complete elimination of fats from the diet. Although many raw foodists have run into problems by eating *too many* avocados, nuts, seeds and oils, it's important not to make the opposite mistake by avoiding them completely.

So I never recommended living on a diet of just fruits and vegetables with no fat sources, and I also never lived on such a diet myself, except for short periods of time when I used it as a cleansing diet.

A Few Words of Advice in Summary

It is human nature when we do something that gives us positive results to think that "more is better." That is why many people who start exercise programs quickly experience fatigue because of over-exercise. With the zeal of the beginner, we take on more than we can handle.

The same happens in the case of diet. People want to lose weight too quickly. They try to cut calories below what is optimal to get faster results, which results in a binge on the rebound.

Similarly, people think, because they feel good going raw, that they'll feel even better by eliminating even more foods from the diet, being stricter, fasting, juice "feasting," and attempting other similar detox diets. Too much of this, like anything else, will sabotage your efforts and create other problems like impaired digestion and social maladjustment.

My suggestion for creating a sustainable maintenance diet rather than a perpetual cleanse, is to stop thinking in terms of "exclusion" and think more in terms of "inclusion."

Instead of always thinking of items you can remove from your diet, think of ways to increase the variety of healthy foods you're eating. Don't limit yourself. Try other things.

It's also especially important to include at least one source of fat in your diet on a regular basis, and avoid going fat-free completely. Eat nuts, seeds, avocados and other fats on a regular basis. Moderation is key, but enjoy these foods regularly. If you find that you can't digest them well anymore, it could be because your overall diet is too strict.

Are Cooked Foods Going to Kill You?

A reader sent me this email:

> This is a very interesting topic and I am eager to read your next book! Sometimes I think that becoming raw was a sort of curse because I have been so brainwashed about the harm of cooked foods that I struggle with even the thought of eating them. And yet I see so many people who could care less about what they eat and they often seem happier and healthier. I would welcome hearing from former raw food fanatics who have changed to a diet with more cooked foods and how the experience has been. After almost 13 years raw I would like to know how my body might react and what steps I could follow to have an easier transition, both physically and mentally. Best of luck, Fred, with your new writings!

One of the biggest challenges experienced by people who have dabbled with raw foodism and other diets is the fear that certain foods they excluded are somewhat "toxic." Raw-foodists in particular entertain this irrational fear of cooking in all its forms, and tend to actually fear cooked foods, or feel extremely guilty when eating them. This fear can be reinforced by negative experiences brought on when reintroducing cooked foods after a period of raw foodism. As we've discussed in a previous chapter, this reintroduction can often lead to digestive issues.

Some people have spent so much time and energy convincing themselves that raw foods are the absolute answer, and that cooked foods are actually toxic, that even when they decide a 100% raw food diet is not right for them, they still feel very uneasy about reintroducing cooked foods. Sometimes, this guilt and fear can even lead to health problems in and of themselves. Combined with a tendency to overanalyze everything that happens in their body (any sign of indigestion, the passing of gas, or a change in body odor) guilt and fear will further increase their neurosis around food.

The problem is that some authors are so convinced that cooked foods are "toxic," they've managed to convince their readers, even when the substance of their argumentation is rather specious.

An objective look at the science will reveal that although cooking food changes its molecular structure, there is no proof that this process is inherently unhealthy. The crux of the matter seems to be *which* foods are eaten, rather than *how* they are cooked. Even though certain cooking methods have definite disadvantages (frying in oil comes to mind), the choice of food is the bigger and more important factor affecting our health.

Raw foodists have used a number of arguments to promote their diet, many of which blame the act of cooking food as a disease-causing agent. To counter all these claims in details would require too much space (perhaps an entire book), and would distract from the main message I'm trying to convey in this one. For those interested in furthering their knowledge, the most complete source of information on the topic I know of is the website **www.beyondveg.com** edited by Tom Billings of San Francisco. Although the website goes in different directions, some of which I don't fully endorse, the section dedicated to the debunking of raw food arguments is absolutely priceless, very well researched, and gives a balanced view on the subject.

The conclusion from all the research available is that raw foodists are not 100% wrong in claiming some forms of cooking are unhealthy, but they are far from being right when they indict all cooked foods as a chief cause of disease.

Some problems with cooking (and how to avoid them)

Cooking at high temperatures can create carcinogens

We know that some methods of food preparation can be harmful no matter what the food is. High-heat cooking is a good example. Exposure of food to high heat may be convenient, quick, and smell great, but it comes at a cost.

There are several unhealthy consequences to high-heat, dry-heat cooking. One is called AGEs, which stands for "advanced glycation end products," a group of chemicals produced by a chain reaction following the combination of a protein molecule with a sugar molecule. A hallmark of AGEs is browning or caramelization.

Foods containing AGEs cause more tissue damage and inflammation than foods cooked at lower temperatures, or raw foods. AGEs irritate cells in the body, damaging tissues and increasing your risk of complications from diseases like diabetes and heart disease. These chemicals can be avoided by cooking meals at lower temperatures using other, wetter cooking methods such as sautéing, steaming, or stir-frying, and also by cooking meats with foods containing antioxidant bioflavonoids, such as garlic, onion, and peppers, and with acidic ingredients such as vinegar or lemon juice.

AGEs are formed in greater quantities from cooking meat in the presence of sugar than from cooking grains or vegetables, because of the greater amount of protein in meat. They are also deliberately used as additives and flavor enhancers in processed foods, and they can also be produced in the human body as part of its own digestive processes.

Most people are not aware that when you cook meat (whether it's grilled, broiled, or seared) there are compounds that can form called HCAs (heterocyclic amines), which are carcinogenic. [6]

As an aside, when you cook meat in a water base, as opposed to grilling, broiling, or searing, you eliminate the harmful HCAs and reduce AGE formation. So for example, cooking meats in a soup or crockpot will not have the problem of the carcinogenic HCAs, and so these are healthier ways to cook meat.

If you're going to grill meats, marinating them for several hours beforehand in liquid mixtures that contain rosemary and other herbs/spices can dramatically help reduce HCAs.

It appears that the highly potent antioxidants in these herbs prevent HCA formation. So using rosemary, thyme, garlic, oregano, and other spices in a marinade before grilling meats can drastically reduce any carcinogens that would normally form on grilled meat and give you a healthier meal that also tastes great.

One more important point about grilling meat.

Remember that the more meat is cooked, the higher the concentration of carcinogenic HCAs formed, so rare, medium-rare, or medium are healthier choices than well done.

---

6   Two separate types of carcinogenic compounds are produced by high-temperature grilling:

* **heterocyclic amines (HCAs)**

    HCAs form when a meat is directly exposed to a flame or very high-temperature surface. The creatine-rich meat juices react with the heat to form various HCAs, including amino-imidazo-quinolines, amino-imidazo-quinoxalines, amino-imidazo-pyridines, and aminocarbolines. HCAs have been shown to cause DNA mutation, and may be a factor in the development of certain cancers.

* **polycyclic aromatic hydrocarbons (PAHs)**

    PAHs form in smoke that's produced when fat from the meat ignites or drips on the hot coals of the grill. Various PAHs present in the resulting smoke, including benzo[a]pyrene and dibenzo[a,h]anthracene, adhere to the outside surface of the grilled meat. PAH exposure is also believed to be linked to certain cancers.

Also, even charring vegetables on the grill creates different carcinogens such as acrylamides, so don't think that the negative effect of charring only applies to meats.

Cooking concentrates calories

Probably the most obvious problem with cooking, which is only a problem in the modern world, is that it predigests foods and therefore makes the calories more available. This gave humans a survival advantage over other animals through the eons we've evolved on this planet. However, in today's world where food is too easily available and often very rich in calories, a diet composed mainly of cooked foods can be a problem. As we've seen in earlier chapters, some whole foods, even when cooked, still have a low caloric density. This includes whole grains, beans, and all vegetables. If you base your diet on these whole foods, avoid refined foods (like flour) and eat plenty of raw foods, you will be able to maintain your weight even when eating cooked foods.

Cooking fats and oils can oxidize them and render them toxic or carcinogenic.

Cooking fats can be a problem, especially the unstable oils such as polyunsaturated fats (especially the delicate oils in fish, and oil-rich plant foods such as nuts, and oils extracted from them). Monounsaturated fats like those in olives and avocados are somewhat resistant to oxidation, and saturated fats like coconut oil are the most resistant of all, even at high heat. But just as you don't want a salad saturated in oil because it massively increases the calories without signaling a person to eat less of it, the same applies to cooking with oil. The solution is to avoid cooking with fat most of the time, and instead, add fats after foods have been cooked.

Some advantages to cooking

Increases nutritional variety

It's simply possible to eat more foods if you cook. Many vegetables, although technically edible raw, are too rich in fiber to be enjoyed without being softened with heat. For example, artichokes are not particularly appealing raw. Cooking allows us to access a wider variety of foods, and ultimately a wider variety of nutrient sources.

Cooking makes foods easier to digest

As we've seen, this can actually be a problem in the modern world, but in many cases it's a boon. Research has shown that cooking makes most foods much easier to digest, particularly protein and starches. The appropriate amount of raw foods versus cooked foods in your diet depends on your goals. If you need to lose weight, increase the percentage of raw fruits and vegetables, especially low-calorie ones (almost all raw vegetables are very low in calories). If you lead a very active lifestyle and burn a lot of calories, or you desire to gain muscle mass, increase the percentage of cooked food in your diet and total calories coming from all macronutrients (protein, fat, carbohydrates).

In the context of a diet that contains a fair amount of raw foods, cooking food does not represent a true health risk. If certain cooking methods are avoided, such as frying or grilling, and healthy foods are consumed, then cooking some food is truly a non-issue.

Alternatives to a 100% Raw Diet

Many people who experiment with raw diets realize they are not going to follow this diet at a 100% level in the long term, or they are not getting the results they desire on the program. Even many low-fat raw vegans (those who eat plenty of fruit to meet their caloric needs, green vegetables, and little fat) also eventually feel that way.

We've already covered the reasons that can lead someone to be attracted to a raw food diet, but also why a 100% raw food diet is not appropriate for most people.

So many ex-raw foodists end up "shopping" other diets and pick one that is more likely to meet their needs.

Going from a low-fat raw vegan diet to a low-fat cooked vegan diet is a natural choice. In fact, the philosophy of the low-fat raw vegan diet was actually "imported" from the low-fat vegan movement.

Nowadays, almost no serious health author uses the word "vegan," to avoid the associations people have with that word and also to distance themselves from the ethical vegans, who often make inferior diet choices. The term "plant-based diet" or "low-fat plant-based diet" is used to describe the program instead.

This philosophy is espoused by many serious health writers — mostly doctors — and varies from one author to the next. Here are the main differences in these philosophies:

Author	Foods Allowed	Forbidden Foods	Restricted Foods
John McDougall (The McDougall Diet)	Grains, beans, vegetables. Salt is allowed.	Meat, fish, eggs, oils — and all animal products except on special occasions	Fruits: 3 pieces a day Nuts, seeds, avocados, tofu, and other higher fat foods: allowed in smaller quantities for those with no weight problems. Restricted or eliminated in weight loss plans. Flour, white rice, and unlimited servings of grains or pasta: allowed for most people; restricted or eliminated in weight loss version of the program
Dr. Caldwell Esselstyn (Heart Attack-Proof)	Grains, beans, vegetables, Fruit Alcohol allowed Coffee, tea allowed	"Anything that has a mother or a face" — all animal products are eliminated. Also eliminated completely: all oils, nuts, seeds, avocados, coconut products, and soy products (because they are high in fat); refined flour, refined grains	Flax seeds every day for omega-3 Walnuts for those who don't have heart disease Smoothies, juices not allowed Fruit restricted to 3 pieces a day for most people, salt restricted or eliminated
Dr. Caldwell Esselstyn (Heart Attack-Proof)	Grains, beans, vegetables, Fruit Alcohol allowed Coffee, tea allowed	"Anything that has a mother or a face" — all animal products are eliminated. Also eliminated completely: all oils, nuts, seeds, avocados, coconut products, and soy products (because they are high in fat); refined flour, refined grains	Flax seeds every day for omega-3 Walnuts for those who don't have heart disease Smoothies, juices not allowed Fruit restricted to 3 pieces a day for most people, salt restricted or eliminated

All of the programs above generally get less than 10% of total calories from fat, although in some cases up to 15% is allowed. The Dr. Fuhrman *Eat to Live* program is quite different and will be covered separately.

These diets are very effective programs for preventing and reversing heart disease, and although they are strict (with the Esselstyn program being the strictest), good results can be expected.

Raw foodists are generally attracted to these programs as alternatives to a raw vegan diet because of the similarity in philosophy. Some authors like John McDougall have created different versions of their diet, one being more appropriate for weight loss and the other less strict, for maintenance.

Overall, from what I have observed having attended the live conferences, people following these programs are generally much older than the raw food crowd and have lots of existing medical conditions.

The problems that seem to plague raw foodists—excessive weight loss, dental decay, failure to thrive, etc.—are not observed on these programs.

The one thing I have noticed, however, is that these programs are all very effective for sustained weight loss, but a "plateau" is often reached, beyond which it is very difficult to lose more weight unless complex carbs are significantly reduced and vegetable intake is increased.

These programs have been designed for sick individuals; therefore they are rarely appropriate, unmodified, for an active, athletic person. For younger, more athletic people who burn lots of calories daily, it would be necessary to increase the fat content of the diet for sustained energy.

I've also noticed that because of the absence of fat, some people on these diets often feel unsatisfied even after eating large amounts of food, and will be looking for something else. Generally more fruit will be consumed to compensate, which, in combination with the high starchy carb intake, can lead to weight gain.

When I was "shopping" alternatives to the 100% raw food lifestyle, I eventually followed the McDougall program for a while. But I have since then modified it to include more raw foods (including daily smoothies), less starch, more beans, more fruit, and a somewhat higher fat intake than would be normally "allowed" on these programs — in addition to not sticking to a 100% vegan diet, as I mentioned previously. My own diet is more appropriate for my age and activity level.

Fuhrman Eat to Live

Dr. Fuhrman's *Eat to Live* program is also very popular, although more complex and difficult to follow than some of the other low-fat vegan alternatives. It is actually quite different from, let's say, the McDougall Diet, so it deserves a category of its own.

The main differences are Fuhrman's insistence on "nutrient density," a higher fat intake, a higher intake of vegetables, and the restriction of certain complex carbs like potatoes. Also, Fuhrman allows a certain percentage of animal products in the diet, although most people following his program are vegans.

Allowed foods: Raw vegetables, cooked vegetables (especially greens), fresh fruit, beans. Fuhrman actually advises that people strive to eat one pound of raw and one pound of cooked vegetables every day, mostly greens. He not only allows fruit but encourages at least 4 pieces a day, or more. He advises eating one cup of beans a day. He encourages eating mushrooms.

Limited: In his weight loss programs, starchy vegetables and whole grains are allowed but greatly limited. But active people can have more

Other foods: 1-2 ounces of nuts a day is advised, or just 1 ounce for weight loss. Flax seeds intake is encouraged. Avocados are encouraged, but limited for weight loss.

Forbidden: Animal food (except if you can limit yourself to less than 12 ounces a week), Dried fruits, except for flavoring, Salt, except maybe 500 mg. a day of added sodium. Oils are excluded, except for active individuals.

The Fuhrman program, being more rounded and less restrictive in some ways, works for a lot of people, but is more difficult to follow than, say, the McDougall Diet. The program is actually more complex than my quick summary, dealing a lot with the concept of nutrient density and seeking foods with the highest ratios. Fuhrman also feels strongly that the McDougall program is too low in fat and too high in carbs to be healthy for most people.

I personally have found great ideas from both Dr. Fuhrman and someone like John McDougall. My own amalgam includes ideas from both parties, together, of course, with principles of raw food nutrition.

The Real Alternative:
The Raw Freedom Program

Ultimately, diets have been designed by authors who appeal to a certain market: people with heart disease, overweight and sick older individuals, or active athletes. If you find that one of these programs targets exactly your situation, then I encourage you to give it a try. Otherwise, you can design your own program based on your needs and current circumstances. Eating shouldn't always be about following "someone's program" but rather choosing the healthiest foods that meet your personal needs.

Now, What Do I Eat?

So far we've covered many important topics, such as when raw food diets are and aren't appropriate for various people and circumstances. We've also seen how to rebuild digestion after following an overly restricted diet for a long period of time.

Now, if you're reading this book, it means you're probably someone who's interested in the benefits that you can gain from various disciplines such as raw foods, periodic fasting, and a plant-based diet.

But this is not a diet book.

I will not impose my way of eating on you and tell you that *this is the only way to eat.*

I also won't just say *eat what works for you* because that's a little vague. This book so far has gone way beyond generic *just eat what works for you*-type advice.

Different Options

A few options are now available to you. You can choose one of them or create your own unique plan.

Your diet plan *will* be healthy, but will also work in your own life circumstances, which are unique to you.

Now, I'm not going to claim that there are different types of diet, for example low-carb or high-carb, and one of them will be right for you.

Rather, what I'm saying is that the general principles of a health diet will apply to everybody, but the actual design of the diet will be different from one person to the next.

Here are some factors that can influence you.

Your past experiences

Your history with diet and nutrition may affect which diet is most appropriate for you. Perhaps you're someone who's been on a never-ending quest to find good health for years and you've jumped from one extreme to the next. In this case, you're just looking to find some balance. Or perhaps you've abused your body too much by unhealthy eating, so that you need something that will give you fast and sustained results.

Your personality

This has more to do with your ability to stick with a strict diet. Are you a consistent and stable person who tends to find one thing and then stick to it forever? Or are you more a "scanner" personality who tends to have many different passions in life and move back and forth from one to the next? Belonging to the latter, I find that I should avoid any statement that resembles "I'm going to do this program for the rest of my life."

Your health

Weaker digestions will need a blander and simpler diet, and also in some cases avoid large quantities of raw vegetables. Those needing to overcome an important health problem quickly may want to consider a stricter version of a plant-based diet, higher on the raw side. Athletes will be mostly concerned with caloric and nutrient-density.

Your personal intolerances

What foods tend to drag you down the most? What do you react most negatively to? What do you have trouble digesting? All of these personal sensitivities can be taken into account.

Your weight goals

Generally speaking, the more weight you have to lose, the more "raw" your diet should be. Athletes needing to maintain their weight should look at a combination of raw and cooked foods. Finally, underweight individuals should increase the percentage of healthy, caloric-dense cooked foods in their diet and not attempt to live on a 100% raw food diet.

Your activity level

If you're relatively sedentary, a very high-raw diet can work well. For active individuals, a raw diet only works when it includes absurd amounts of fruit. More realistically, if you go through a lot of calories during the day and have trouble getting them in, you need to add more cooked foods and healthy fats to your diet.

Your ethics

The vegan/animal rights issue is a touchy one for diet choice. Some feel very strongly about it, either being totally for or against it. Generally, people quit the vegan diet having decided it wasn't the *healthiest* approach for them. Strict vegans tend to be more motivated by *ethical* reasons. Either way, the *raw freedom* approach can work for you.

Your location

A warmer climate is indeed more conducive to a raw food diet. Availability of produce can also be an issue, although in most big cities of the world it is not a problem — and in fact has never been better. Many people I know who live in Northern countries tend to eat a higher-raw diet in the summer and incorporate more cooked foods in the winter.

Your job

Do you travel a lot for business? Does your occupation require that you attend many events where food is served, or meet clients for lunch or dinner? Finding the right compromise in such cases is very important. In fact, they should not just be viewed as "compromises" but as part of your overall lifestyle.

Your lifestyle

Some people never travel abroad. Others, like me, can't help but get on a plane a few times a year and spend time in foreign countries. I already determined a while ago that trying to maintain a raw food diet (or even a strict vegan diet) while traveling takes much of the fun out of traveling. With that conclusion, I made sure that my diet allows enough flexibility for the weeks of the year when I'm traveling.

For all the above reasons, there's no diet that will be 100% right for everybody. Don't be ashamed of the option that works for you. A diet can de designed to be perfectly healthy and still allow enough flexibility for you to enjoy eating out, eating cooked foods, and even eating occasional "junk." What matters is what you do most of the time.

Also, cooked foods are not unhealthy. Rather, it's the type of cooking that makes the difference, the use of refined ingredients, and what foods are being cooked. If you have been trying to live up to the raw food ideal, it is important to get rid of this silly notion that all cooked foods are unhealthy.

What Percentage is Right for You?

A reader writes:

I don't think any sort of fixed ratio is "best." Learning to tune into intuitive guidance and release any guilt, shame or fear is what I try to do. I often find that I am guided to eat sugary foods when I am experiencing a creative block. The "sugar high" helps me to break through my inhibitions. Yes, I pay for it, but I am also rewarded by the ability to express myself. Health is more than just physical.

Eat 100% Raw

Eating 100% raw is certainly not for everybody, but there's no doubt it works for some people, at least for a while. But these people would like to convince you that their diet works for everybody. Most people I know who claim they eat 100% raw upon closer examination cheat on their diet a few times a year. But in all honesty, we can still consider them raw foodists because they are very close to eating their intended diet. A few cheat meals once in a while don't really count overall.

A 100% raw diet can be used as a cure or a sort of detox diet. It can be used also to lose weight. A few things to keep in mind when eating 100% raw:

- Make sure you track your calories to ensure you're eating enough
- Don't neglect the few necessary supplements that every vegan and raw foodist needs, such as B12
- Consume at least one pound of raw greens a day, if not more. Try to make green smoothies and other blended recipes to make it easier for you to consume those greens.
- Get most of your calories from fruit, and restrict the fat. However, don't cut out fat completely. Get about 15% of your calories from fat (including nuts and seeds). A raw low-fruit diet works for very few people because it's too low in calories and energy.

- Pay particular attention to dental health, and go for a checkup every six months instead of yearly, to make sure no problem pops up.

I suspect that very few people reading this book will actually eat a 100% raw food diet. It's not a plan that can appeal to a lot of people; certainly not one that can be enthusiastically recommended for everyone in every phase of life.

Eat 75% raw

A good alternative to a pure raw food diet is the 75 or 80% raw diet. This is a diet where you essentially eat most of your food raw, but have a little something cooked every day to help you get your calories and meet your nutrient needs.

Certain cooked foods are actually very nutritious and I can't think of a circumstance where it wouldn't be beneficial to eat them regularly. Beans and cooked greens particularly come to mind.

The key with the 75% raw diet is not to fall into the trap of making this a 100% raw diet with an occasional cooked meal. As we've seen, your digestive system will adapt to the foods you eat on a regular basis. You should pick a side—either eat cooked foods regularly, or leave them out. Otherwise, you risk the digestive problems and other woes described in chapter XX.

So if you choose to eat 75% raw, eat some cooked foods every day, or 4-5 times a week. At that level, the best cooked foods to eat would be:

- Cooked sweet potatoes, and other root vegetables.
- Beans (legumes, etc.)
- Cooked vegetables of all kinds (artichokes, asparagus, kale, etc.)
- Lean animal protein (fish, etc.)

At the 75% level, it's best to choose cooked foods that will complement your overall nutritional profile, rather than fall into the trap of eating massive amounts of cooked carbs (bread, white pasta, etc.) to fill the caloric void. Make sure you get calories from both raw and cooked foods.

By the way, this level of raw food eating is a good target for most people reading this book. If you have trouble maintaining your weight or if you have a significant amount of weight to lose, then shooting for a high percentage of raw food makes sense. One exception would be for people with very sensitive digestion who can't handle a lot of raw fiber, as well as those who find that their energy significantly drops when eating a high-raw diet.

Eat "A lot" of Raw 50%

The next level is not really a raw food diet. This is where you incorporate elements of the raw food lifestyle (green smoothies, big raw salads, blended salads, fruit meals, etc.) into a balanced diet that includes raw and cooked foods. Your goal is not to aim at a particular percentage. Your goal is just to be healthy.

This is a good level to aim at for people wanting to clean up their diet, for most men, and for active people already at their ideal weight. This is where I personally stand. I don't try to count the percentage of raw food in my diet anymore. Sometimes it's high, sometimes it's not. I make adjustments as I go along.

Not a Raw Food Diet at All

Finally, some people will find it better and healthier to completely get out of the concept of eating a high-raw diet. In this case, you don't eat a raw diet. Most of the food you eat will be cooked, but every day you will have a few pieces of fruit and hopefully a big salad. Most of your calories will come from cooked food, but some of the bulk will come from raw foods.

This level would be advisable for severely underweight people with digestive issues. These people shouldn't attempt a raw food diet. Most of the food they eat should be high in calories, and I would advise eating some refined foods that are extremely digestible such as white rice and even white bread, along with a good amount of healthy fats (nut butters, for example).

Some people simply don't have the time or desire to eat a lot of raw food. Or maybe they tried and it didn't work. For example, up until about two years ago, my mom was carrying a lot of excess weight. I always tried to help her go on a diet, and she even went raw for a month. But nothing worked. So I suggested she try a simple diet containing only whole grains, beans, vegetables, and some fruit. The main food she ate during that time was oatmeal, along with big plates of vegan chili with brown rice. She lost 55 pounds in 8-9 months and never put it back on.

Traps

The foods we eat on a daily basis form habits. If you eat a raw food diet, you will eventually get used to a raw food diet and it will feel normal to eat this way.

Because cooked foods can be very convenient, it can be easy to fall into the trap of eating too many cooked and prepared foods and let good habits like consuming large salads, fruit, green juices, and smoothies fall by the wayside. Suddenly your 60 or 70% raw diet becomes a 10% raw diet, and it's hard to get back on track.

The key to avoiding this is to keep the good habits going. And you do that by making an effort to eat raw foods *first*. Since making a big salad is extra work when you're already cooking something, you won't feel like doing it after you've cooked up your meal and you're hungry. So eat the salad *first* and then have your cooked food. Or prepare the salad first and only add the other foods once the salad is ready.

Juicing is easier if you do it first thing in the morning. Juice extracted with a good juicer will keep fresh for the better part of a day.

Smoothies are easy to make, but eating enough fruit takes some organization. You have to make sure you have ripe fruit available, and go shopping often to avoid running out.

The easiest way to make sure your diet is balanced in the direction that you want is to have a *pattern* of eating. We'll discuss this more when we look at various menu plans you can put together.

Vegan or not?

As part of the cooked foods you can eat, animal foods may come to mind. This book won't tell you that you have to be vegan or not. However, there are many ways to have some freedom in this department. Some people like a *flexitarian* approach where they eat a near-vegan diet most of the time, but occasionally "cheat," especially for special occasions or while traveling. Others prefer to stick to a vegan diet all the time, while others will feel best with some lean animal products on a regular basis. We've already discussed that it's possible to eat some animal products as part of your diet and overall create a very healthy diet. It's also possible to stay vegan and be healthy.

Most health experts agree that a plant-based diet is best. Ketogenic diets that emphasize animal products can be just as extreme as overly restricted raw vegan diets. Keeping animal products to a relative minimum is a good idea, but the choice of animal products to be eaten is probably the most important factor. The animal products that can provide the most benefits are:

- Fish rich in omega-3 fats (wild salmon, rainbow trout, red snapper, etc.)
- Other fish from "clean" and sustainable sources (in some cases, farmed fish is best, in some, wild fish is best).
- Low-fat, fermented dairy products (yogurt, etc.), but not including cheese.
- 100% grass-fed meat or grain-fed fowl from organic sources.
- Eggs, eaten occasionally and in moderation.

Many theories abound regarding animal products, and some people advocate going "full-fat" and not fearing the cholesterol content of eggs or butter. Feel free to believe what you want, but the scientific consensus is that the saturated fat content of animal products, as well as its cholesterol content, is one of the main factors in the development of heart disease. In some cases, animal products can be very low in saturated fat. A fillet of fish contains almost no saturated fat, compared to high amounts in some plant foods.

Some people are genetically prone to heart disease and will react strongly to the cholesterol and saturated fat content of foods. Therefore, it's important to monitor yourself through yearly blood tests and make adjustments if necessary.

I do believe that a low-fat, exclusively plant-based diet can be a great choice for a great number of people because of its healing properties. But I also think that a moderate inclusion of animal products in the diet can be healthy; and more importantly, can add an element of freedom in certain social situations or simply add variety to the overall diet and avoid boredom.

A Raw Food Lunch, or Not

The easiest way to eat more raw food and get closer to the 70% mark (if that's the goal) is to consume a raw food lunch in addition to a raw food breakfast. If you've determined that your body type would do better with a higher-raw diet, then make sure that you don't consume any cooked food until dinner. Breakfast is easy, and can be a green smoothie. But make sure you don't make the mistake of only having a big salad with no cooked carbs or protein for lunch. Such a salad (composed of vegetables and raw fat sources) is not very sustaining for most people, except those with extremely low caloric needs. So go for more fruit, in addition to the salad — or fruit only (either alone, in smoothies, or in green smoothies) for your lunch meal, if you decide to make it raw.

A Stable Routine Is Best

Eating in the same fashion, day after day, is best for overall health and stability. This doesn't mean you'll eat the same foods at every meal, but that the general *pattern* of your diet will be consistent. For example, it's best to have more or less the same percentage of raw food every day, so your body can adapt. If you have a 100% raw day on Monday and then eat 80% cooked food on Tuesday, you will confuse your body. So stick to a routine, and make modifications along the way.

Designing Your Own Raw-Based Program

Going from an "exclusion" to an "inclusion" mindset means you'll think more about what you're eating than about what you're avoiding. You want to keep some freedom to eat the cooked foods that you enjoy, but also keep a strong *raw* element in the program. For some people, this will mean eating the majority of their food raw. For others, a 50% approach is best. Finally, some people will do best eating most of their calories cooked, but keep some raw foods for nutritional purposes. The three types have been discussed elsewhere in the book.

Raw Habits to Include

Every raw eating habit is a discipline that can require some time to establish. If you find it too difficult to incorporate all of these disciplines at the same time start with one, and then move on to another once the first discipline is firmly established.

The Daily Green Smoothie

By far the easiest raw food habit that gives the most positive results for most people is the green smoothie habit. A green smoothie is simply a blended drink made with a liquid (usually water, but I like to use oil-free, store-bought almond milk as well), fruit (ripe bananas and another type of fruit are usually part of the mix), and a good amount of raw, green vegetables (baby spinach, de-stemmed kale, celery, and lettuce leaves of all types are usually the main greens). This smoothie is chock-full of nutrition and if you include enough fruit, it can be very sustaining. Many people report amazing benefits just from adopting that habit! I personally often add a scoop of raw protein powder to the green smoothie, since I've been weight-lifting more intensely.7 Green smoothies can be an ideal breakfast, but also a lunch! Some people like to only sustain themselves on green smoothies and cut-up fruit during the day, and report feeling amazing that way.

Green Vegetable Juices

Juicing is more of a discipline than making green smoothies. It takes a bit more effort to prepare the vegetables, juice them, and wash the juicer. However, reasonable quantities of green juice can be extremely beneficial for health. The minerals and nutrients extracted in a low-heat juicer are easily absorbable and can significantly enhance your health. It's okay to use a bit of carrot or apple to sweeten your juice, but the base should be green. My favorite juice includes 2 carrots, several sticks of celery; spinach or kale, one small apple, Romaine lettuce, half a small beet, one inch of ginger, and lemon.

---

7   Although I talked about protein powders negatively in the past, some new products have recently been developed that meet my approval. They can be useful for people who choose to eat a very restricted raw food diet, or people like me who see benefits in terms of satiety and muscle gain results from adding a scoop of such powders in a daily green smoothie. I started lifting weights more intensely in November 2012 and have since then gained over 12 pounds of muscle. My favorite products are made by Sunwarrior and Growing Naturals, and use sprouted brown rice as a main ingredient.

Eating a Lot of Fruit

Fruit is extremely healthy, and yet it's commonly vilified in natural health circles, or recommended only in "strict moderation." The fructose in fruit is often blamed and even equated to refined fructose that is overly abundant in the American diet and at the root of many health problems. Fruit is inherently healthy because of the fiber it contains, but also because it doesn't contain just one type of sugar, but many. Some sugars are absorbed immediately (like glucose), some are absorbed more slowly (like fructose), and others are bound with fiber and digested in the small intestine. Because of this, fruit is lower on the glycemic index than most grains, and an extremely good source of sustained energy. However, if you do eat a lot of fruit, you will consume a lot of natural sugar. This is not a problem if you are in good health and can process sugars efficiently as a result of good lifestyle habits. If you eat more fruit, you automatically have to reduce the quantity of cooked starch in your diet. Otherwise, large quantities of fruit combined with good or large quantities of starches will lead to extra energy and weight gain. Also, since low-fat diets improve insulin sensitivity and the ability to process sugar efficiently, the more fruit you consume, the lower in fat your diet should be. Most people eating normal quantities of fruit (a few pieces a day) and the rest of their calories from starches, protein and fat could consume up to 30% fat in their diet without seeing too many problems in sugar assimilation. But as you eat more fruit, the fat percentage in your diet should be lower. That's why people who live almost exclusively on fruit have to almost avoid all fats—otherwise the combination of a high-sugar diet with a high-fat diet could lead to serious insulin-related problems. In general, a fat consumption of around 20% combined with an above-average fruit consumption is quite okay. Combined with physical activity and a good diet, you should have no problem handling the extra sugar in fruit. As I've mentioned, this sugar cannot be equated to refined sugar in any way.

Some individuals will find it better to temporarily dramatically lower or even almost eliminate fruit from their diet. Raw foodists who have experienced a streak of dental decay on a fruit-based diet, and raw vegans who have wrecked and weakened their digestion through an overly restricted diet, combined with an excessive consumption of acid fruits (like oranges and pineapple) would be advised to give their body a much needed respite from fruit for a few weeks and up to a few months. During that time, most of your calories will come from healthy starches, as well as some fat and protein. All of the vitamins in fruits can be found in raw vegetables, so there is no danger or negative to temporary complete removal of fruit from the diet.

The Daily Big Salad

This discipline is best adopted for dinner time, but is one that I personally have trouble integrating due to the fact that my weight-training regimen leaves me very hungry most of the day. I always feel like I *must* eat when it's dinner time, and often skip the time and energy necessary to make and eat a big salad. That's why I try to get more of my vegetables through green smoothies and juicing.

The Blended Salad

This daily habit is just as good as a big salad, but takes less time and can be a solution for people who just can't seem to manage the cutting and chewing required for a big salad.

A blended salad is *not* a green smoothie. But the concept is similar. The key is to include the following ingredients:

- Tomatoes, cucumbers, and other "soft" and mild-tasting vegetables
- Greens of your choice (usually lettuce and spinach)
- Celery
- Something sweet (like mango, or a sweetener like honey)

- Something to give taste (fresh herbs, garlic, green onions, scallions, hot peppers, etc.)

It's possible to replace the "sweet" element of a blended salad with something fatty, like half an avocado. But my favorite blended salad is light and a little fruity. I pack in a lot of greens.

The key is to avoid blending everything to a complete mush like you would a smoothie. Instead, use the low setting on your blender. You can also add diced veggies to your dish after blending to make it more interesting.

Start with the soft vegetables; add in the celery and greens, and the other ingredients in the order listed. If you're interested in incorporating this habit, I recommend Roger Haeske "Savory Veggie Stews" program at **www.veggiestews.com**

Personally, I like to spice up my blended salads with some Tabasco sauce. Just a few drops give a lot of taste, and essentially no added sodium.

Foods That Are Beneficial to Eat Raw

Almost all fruits and vegetables are very beneficial, but certain foods come to mind as having *extra* properties and health benefits, and we should try to include them even more often in our diet:

Apples

Because of the fiber they contain. They're nature's "slimming" food. If you eat a big apple before every meal, you will drop weight and feel better. Research done at Penn State University showed that people who ate an apple 15 minutes before lunching consumed 187 fewer calories in total than people who snacked on nothing beforehand. 8

Pomegranate seeds

Pomegranate seeds are high in antioxidants, and can aid in preventing muscle cramps and lowering cholesterol. Also, they may play an important role in the prevention of heart disease and cancer because they fight cell damage. One pomegranate contains approximately 50% of your recommended daily amount of vitamin C. They also contain pantothenic acid (B5), which is what helps with the muscle cramping and aids in preventing insulin resistance.

Blueberries, and other berries

Keeping up with your blueberry (and other berry) intake is Berry Beneficial!

---

8   http://usatoday30.usatoday.com/news/health/2007-10-23-apple-diet_N.htm

Blueberries have one of the highest antioxidant contents of all fruits, vegetables, spices, and seasonings. Antioxidants are essential to optimizing health by helping to combat the free radicals that can damage cellular structures as well as DNA. These antioxidant properties benefit your nervous system and brain health, and improve your memory.

You can freeze berries without doing damage to their antioxidant properties. This is great news if you can't find fresh berries but can find them in the freezer section of the market.

Also, berries in general are low on the glycemic index (GI). The glycemic index is a commonly used way to identify the potential impact of a food on our blood sugar level once we've consumed and digested that food. In general, foods with a GI of 50 or below are best in regulating our blood sugar. Blueberries, as well as other berries such as blackberries, raspberries, and strawberries, fall in the range of 30-53.

Kale

Some people call kale the "queen of greens." They know that kale is a powerhouse of nutrients, health benefits; and tastes good too.

Kale, also known as borecole, is one of the most nutritious vegetables on the planet. A leafy green, kale is available in curly, ornamental, or dinosaur varieties. It belongs to the Brassica family that includes cruciferous vegetables such as cabbage, collards, broccoli, and Brussels sprouts.

One cup of kale contains 36 calories, 5 grams of fiber, and 15% of the daily requirement of calcium and vitamin B6, 40% of the magnesium requirement, 180% of vitamin A, 200% of vitamin C, and 1,020% of vitamin K. It is also a good source of minerals: copper, potassium, iron, manganese, and phosphorus.

While all vegetables are good for you, eating kale on a regular basis may provide significant health benefits such as cancer protection and lowered cholesterol.

Kale's health benefits are primarily linked to the high concentration of antioxidant vitamins A, C, and K, as well as phytonutrients.

Kale is also rich in the eye health promoting lutein and zeaxanthin compounds.

Besides the beneficial antioxidants, the fiber content of kale binds bile acids and helps lower blood cholesterol levels and reduce the risk of heart disease, especially when kale is cooked instead of raw.

Almonds

Is there a high-fat food that's good for your health? Yes, that's almonds!

Almonds are an ancient food written about in historical texts, including the Bible. Almonds are thought to have originated in regions in western Asia and North Africa. The Romans referred to almonds as the "Greek nut" in reference to the civilization from which they learned to eat them.

The almond that we think of is technically the seed of the fruit of the almond tree, a medium-sized tree that bears fragrant pink and white flowers. Like its cousins, the peach, cherry and apricot trees, the almond tree bears fruits with stone-like seeds (or pits) within. The seed of the almond fruit is what we refer to as the almond nut.

But what are the health benefits of these nuts that would put them on my "beneficial foods" list?

As I mentioned, they are a high-fat food that's good for your health. Almonds are high in monounsaturated fats, the same health-promoting fats found in olive oil. These fats are associated with reduced risks of heart disease.

Almonds' ability to reduce heart disease risk may also be partly due to the antioxidant action of the vitamin E found in almonds. They are also chock-full of magnesium and potassium. When you have enough magnesium in your system your veins and arteries are content and relaxed. This improves the flow of blood, oxygen, and nutrients throughout the body. Studies show that a deficiency of magnesium is not only associated with heart attack but that immediately following a heart attack, lack of sufficient magnesium promotes free radical injury to the heart.

Potassium is a crucial electrolyte involved in nerve transmission and the contraction of all muscles including the heart. It's also essential for maintaining normal blood pressure and heart function. Almonds promote your cardiovascular health by providing 257 mg of potassium and only 0.3 mg of sodium, making almonds an especially good choice in protecting against high blood pressure and atherosclerosis.

Don't just enjoy almonds as a between-meal snack. Spread a little almond butter on your toast or spread it down the center of a stalk of celery. Add a handful of almonds to your salad or chop and use as a topping for pasta, or steamed or sautéed vegetables. When eating foods with a higher glycemic index, including almonds in the meal can help keep your blood sugar under control.

Avocado

Avocados are naturally high in fat, but it is mostly healthy, monounsaturated fat, essential for smooth, youthful skin. They also stimulate production of anti-wrinkle collagen which, together with vitamin E, makes them the best food to eat for a healthy complexion.

But that's not the main reason they appear on this list.

Avocados are packed with essential nutrients, including potassium, B-vitamins and folic acid. They also act as a nutrient booster, which means that when eaten with other foods, avocados enable the body to better absorb cancer-fighting nutrients, such as carotenoids, which are found in vegetables like spinach and carrots.

The potassium in avocados regulates blood pressure and helps guard against heart disease and strokes, as well as aiding digestion and helping the body flush out toxins. It also helps fight fatigue and depression, both of which reduce your ability to concentrate.

The combination of Vitamins B6, C, D, and riboflavin (B2) found in avocados, as well as manganese, helps maintain a strong immune system. They are also a good source of vitamins A and E, which help protect against cancer. Avocados are high in omega-3, which reduces the risk of heart disease, and they contain lecithin, a type of fatty acid crucial for healthy nervous system tissue.

And besides all these benefits, who can live without guacamole?

Green juices

You see me talking about green juices over and over again because drinking green juice is an amazing way to add health and vitality to your life. Dark green leafy vegetables have an abundance of nutrients in them, everything from iron to protein to vitamin C. Although the fiber has been removed, juicing makes these nutrients extremely bio-available to your body.

It's best to drink green drinks on an empty stomach so that the absorption of nutrients is not hindered. In other words, the best time of day to have your juice is in the morning before eating anything else.

Remember to use a variety of greens in your juices and continually rotate the greens you use in order to get a variety of nutrients. It is best to buy your greens organic and local, or grow your greens yourself.

Be creative with your juices, but always make the main ingredient dark green leafy vegetables. Use vegetables that are in season, and experiment with vegetables you have not tried before. There are so many different kinds of leafy vegetables out there, and they all have their own unique taste.

If you are not used to green drinks they may taste bitter to you at first. Adding cucumber, red bell peppers or a green apple will mask that bitterness and make your juice taste very sweet.

Here is a short list of produce to use in your juices:

GREENS (make greens the bulk of your juice)

- kale
- bok choy
- romaine lettuce
- spinach
- parsley
- cilantro
- basil
- dill
- red or green cabbage
- Swiss chard
- rainbow chard
- collard greens
- arugula
- dandelion greens
- carrot greens
- beet greens

OTHER OPTIONS TO ADD TO YOUR JUICE

- celery
- carrots
- apples
- pears

- bell peppers
- cucumbers
- beets
- fennel
- lemon

To add a little zing to your juice, throw a small piece of ginger into the juicer. Ginger is very warming to the body, which makes this a nice addition on a cold day. Experiment and rotate your vegetables, and have fun with green juices!

Raw Onion

Onions contain important phytonutrients known as allyl sulfides. These sulfur-containing phytonutrients are what give the onions so many of their health promoting qualities.

The striking difference in flavor and aroma that exists between cooked and raw onion is largely due to the effect of cooking on the allyl sulfide phytonutrients, since not only do they contribute to the onions' nutritional qualities but they also impart their pungent flavor and aroma.

So we can either eat raw onions to gain the benefits of these phytonutrients, or cook them.

If you're cooking them here are some tips on how to cook onions so as to maximize their sulfur-containing phytonutrient profile.

Slicing, chopping or mincing onions before cooking will enhance their health-promoting properties.

The finer the onion is cut, the more extensive the activation of the sulfur compounds. The stronger the smell and the more they affect your eyes, the more health-promoting nutrients they contain. So the next time you cut your onion, you will have a greater appreciation of its "irritating" effects, knowing that the pungent smell that makes you cry will also make you healthy!

So, to get the most health benefits from onions, let them sit for a minimum of 5 minutes, and optimally for 10 minutes, after cutting, before eating or cooking. This is to ensure the maximum synthesis of the sulfur compounds.

Cook at low or medium heat for short periods (up to 15 minutes). This should not destroy the active phytonutrients since once they are formed, they are fairly stable.

What About Caffeine?

Can caffeine be included in a "raw freedom" program? Most raw food authors will say an emphatic "No." Even I am tempted to join in a hate campaign against caffeine, simply because I have found I am much more sensitive to caffeine than most folks, and have been so all my life.

Caffeine is a drug — a mild one — but a substance that affects the human body. It has side effects, which can be more or less severe depending on the person. And of course, it creates dependency.

When abused, caffeine can be extremely detrimental, causing a wide range of health problems, from depression to backaches. In this case, the word "abuse" cannot be strictly interpreted, because it will depend on each person's tolerance for caffeine, which can also change in different phases of a single person's life.

As I've talked about extensively on my blog, caffeine has always had a strong pull on me. I've battled against it, only to fall back into it some time later.

Nowadays, I allow myself a little caffeine from time to time, when I feel the need. While traveling and overcoming jetlag, caffeine can be a help. Or sometimes, when I want to stimulate myself to complete a challenging workout at the gym, or to finish a work session, I will use some caffeine.

I use the word "caffeine" as a generic term. My preferred sources are green tea and yerba mate, because they give me the fewest side-effects. But I will also have coffee from time to time.

As long as you are aware of what you're doing; of the effects caffeine has on your body, and its side-effects, I believe there can be a place for it in some people who feel the need. For many people who are not too sensitive to caffeine, a daily cup of coffee is a guilty pleasure that will lead to no serious health consequences. As much as I would love to, I know that personally I can't have a daily cup of coffee, or else my health eventually suffers. I mainly experience irritability and symptoms of mild depression, which go away after a few days of abstinence. However, if I have just one cup of coffee (or another caffeine-containing beverage) one day in isolation, it's not enough to affect me negatively. It's accumulation of caffeine in my system over several days that becomes a big problem.

What Does Frederic Think About... Animal Protein?

Like many people, what led me to embark on a raw food diet was my initial conversion to vegetarianism. And like many people, I became a vegetarian in my youth. Not even 18 years old, I came across some vegetarian literature and while not changing overnight, I eventually decided to become a vegetarian.

I wasn't a vegan, though. I still ate yogurt because I couldn't give up dairy, and I ate regularly at the only vegetarian restaurant I knew, but they did use some dairy and eggs.

I skipped the vegan phase and jumped straight into raw foodism. And when I gave up raw foodism as an ideal, I was naturally drawn to the previous diet I knew best, which was mostly vegetarian but not completely vegan.

Over the years, I've tried different approaches and been exposed to both sides of the debate. On the one hand, there's the "plant-based" movement of doctors who recommend a low fat, essentially vegan diet (McDougall, Esselstyn, Barnard, and many others).

Then we have lower-carb diets, with plenty of room in between. Some go further and even design diets that are *based* on animal products.

I won't argue with the concept of the plant-based diet. However, it seems a bit misleading to me that the doctors who recommend a plant-*based* diet are actually promoting a plant-*exclusive* diet. Plant-*based* implies a diet that is composed *mostly* of plants. And I think the scientific evidence we have is strong enough to say this is best for health. However, where the debate still lies is in whether animal products could play a small but maybe important role, in the context of a plant-*based* diet. Most of your calories should still come from plants... but who's to say that a small percentage of calories coming from select animal products couldn't be beneficial?

It's a big debate, and I don't pretend to have all the answers. The gurus are debating it vehemently, and often I think vegan ethics and other bias come in the way of real science. So far, I haven't seen any evidence that getting, let's say, 5-10% of your calories from animal foods would be detrimental for health.

The biggest controversy that this book will generate in the raw food world probably has nothing to do with the debate between raw and cooked food, but rather the use of animal products. In raw foodists circles, veganism has become an even touchier subject than raw versus cooked.

The reason is that most raw foodists happen to be staunch vegans, but on the other hand, some ex-raw foodists have reverted to animal products and actually *speak out* against pure veganism. I find myself in the middle. I don't agree with people who say vegan diets *can't* be healthy, but I also can't agree with vegans who say that 100% veganism is the only way to go and there can't be any health benefits in consuming *some* animal products in your diet if you so desire.

There are many emotions attached to this issue, which made me hesitant to say much about it in this book. However, I realized I had to talk about it because, in my personal case, giving up on the *vegan* ideal was just as important as giving up on the raw food ideal.

As you will discover, I remain committed to a plant-*based* diet, and am not one of those people who feel it's absolutely necessary for health to include animal foods in the diet. However, for a number of reasons, I prefer not to be a strict vegan.

My main reasons for doing so are:

- I now prefer to be more *inclusive* than *exclusive*. And it seems odd to me to want to exclude an entire category of food (animal products) that has played an important part in human nutrition for probably as long as we've been around on this planet.

- I find it easier not to be a strict vegan, for social reasons.
- I enjoy the added variety of being able to consume *some* animal products.
- I actually think there are some health benefits to consuming *some* animal products; I haven't seen my health degrade in any way from consuming them in small but regular quantities. In fact, my digestion is much better, and my energy more balanced.

There's nothing inherently wrong with a strict diet — vegan or raw — as long as it is nutritionally balanced, works for you, and you are happy with it.

The raw food diet, in its purest form, is probably one of the strictest diets ever designed. The low-fat, natural hygiene version of the raw food diet is even stricter. Only raw fruits, vegetables, nuts and seeds must be consumed, with no condiments or seasonings.

Compared to a raw food diet, a *vegan* diet that allows cooked foods appears to be quite permissive. After all, there's an entire world of foods that must be cooked to be enjoyed, and can still be considered vegan. Beans, grains, and many vegetables all fall in this category. And if seasonings are permitted, these foods can all be prepared in many creative ways.

However, only a raw foodist would see a vegan diet as a permissive diet. Coming from the prison of raw foods, going to a vegan diet is like going from high level security to low level security detention. But to many other people, it would still be a prison!

Having traveled all around the world, I know for a fact that a raw food diet is impossible to maintain, but even just a cooked vegan diet can also very difficult to maintain while traveling. The reason is that not a single major culture in the world is vegan. Although many cultures eat dramatically smaller quantities of animal products than we do in the West, you'd be hard pressed to find many dishes that are actually vegan.

For example, in Thailand, fish sauce is used in almost everything. It actually gives the flavor many people associate with Thai food. Trying to order Thai food that's truly vegan would be like trying to order cooked food made without heat!

I understand that there are ethical arguments for not eating animal products. I think every reader will be able to determine where she stands on this issue. In any case, I still recommend sourcing animal products from sustainable and clean sources.

In terms of health, no one has all the answers, but I think there are interesting arguments to look at on both sides of the fence. It's fairly clear that a rich diet containing, among other things, a lot of animal products, is not conducive to health. But this issue is not black and white. Although some people do believe that the ideal human diet is a sort of "paleo" diet where animal products predominate, actual evidence does not support this theory.

In terms of health, the real question is: *Can you get some benefits from eating animal products, and if so, what is the upper limit?*

As is the case with other foods, animal products should be consumed in a certain context. For example, avocados are great for health. But should you eat three to five avocados a day like some raw foodists do? Of course not. That would be far too much fat and calories. So for most people, half an avocado a day is the right amount. In addition, avocados won't be your sole source of fat. Other days, you might consume nuts, or maybe a bit of olive oil.

Before we get into the health aspects of eating animal products, let me finish off with the psychological or social reasons for not being vegan.

My Process and Why I Stopped Being Vegan

In *Raw Food Controversies*, I described how I lost my vegan idealism after experiencing a streak of absolute dental decay on a raw vegan diet. My teeth were on the verge of falling apart from rampant decay, and I had to do something. So I stopped being raw, and I stopped being vegan. As I explained, not only did I put a complete end to the decay; I also reversed some existing cavities (in their early stages, but would have grown to full-blown cavities if not prevented).

That visit to the dentist was where my entire vegan idealism disappeared. And it has never come back since.

In all of my books since then, I made it clear that I was not a vegan and that I occasionally experimented with animal products. However, I also stated that my preference was to eat a plant-based diet, and that I rarely consumed animal products.

Of course I have wanted to explore this issue more, because I find the debate fascinating.

One of the ways the body and mind are altered after long periods on a raw food diet is through deprivation of food variety, and also having developed the habit of eating large quantities of low-calorie foods in order to thrive.

So when a raw foodist goes from an all or mostly raw food diet to a cooked food diet, it's often very difficult for him to adjust to the change.

After many months or years of eating only a small variety of foods and restricting yourself to certain tastes, deciding to eat cooked food is like being a hungry kid in a candy store. You want to eat and try everything, and can stuff yourself enough to make yourself sick. On top of that, your digestion can be pretty weak after many years of eating raw, so that your body can't handle everything you're throwing its way.

But in certain circumstances, it seems, the body can handle pretty much any food you give it.

In 2006, I was fairly close to 100% raw. I ate a high-fruit diet, kept my fat intake to a minimum, drank huge banana smoothies for lunch, and only ate cooked foods a few times a month. And even those cooked foods would be fairly similar each time.

During that year I was in Costa Rica, in a very stressful situation. I had decided to purchase and run a retreat center with a girlfriend who was also my business partner. The project was a really bad financial decision, and getting it off the ground was very difficult. On top of that, my girlfriend became mentally ill over the course of several months. Her illness turned into a full-blown psychosis that wasn't resolved for many weeks. Before the actual psychotic episode, her mental instability was extremely taxing for everyone around her. Living with someone who's mentally ill, especially when you don't know what they're suffering from and can't even convince them they have a problem, is a horrible experience I couldn't have imagined without going through it. Handling someone going through full-blown psychosis is a truly traumatizing experience I don't wish on anyone.

That year, I was in hell.

The business was going down, my partner was going crazy, the entire project we started together was going under; and on top of that we were living in a third-world country, with no easy access to family members who could help or advise us.

At some point during that adventure, something happened to me.

I tried to make my usual banana smoothie, and I almost gagged. I just could not eat another banana smoothie. The thought of it was repulsive to me.

It happened overnight. One day, I was consuming my fruit meals and my smoothies and salad. The next day, I couldn't look at those same foods.

I was craving *food*. In a big way. By *food* I mean real, stick-to-your-bones, heavy duty, sustaining meals my lumberjack grandfather would have recognized as food.

So I started by eating a plate of rice and beans, the national dish of Costa Rica.

The next day, I was craving more. So I ate more rice and beans.

I was also craving coffee, so I started drinking it every day.

After about a week, I added some eggs, which Costa Ricans usually eat with their rice and beans in the morning.

After a while, I was eating everything. I had a huge appetite. I started eating bread, and meat too. I ate fish, and chicken, and beef, and lamb. And at every meal, I would go back for second helpings. In fact, I ate such a large quantity of foods that most people told me I was actually eating two or three times the quantity that a normal adult would be eating. I also drank beer and wine.

Because most of our workers at the retreat center were not raw foodists or even vegetarian, we got in the habit of preparing a big meal every night to feed everybody that would content both the vegetarians and the meat-eaters.

The strangest thing was that throughout that whole time, my digestion was great. My sleep was great. And considering the incredible amount of stress I was under, just the fact that I could fall asleep at night was a miracle in itself.

I kept up this new diet for several months until the entire project went under, my girlfriend became really sick, and we all went back to Canada. Our relationship fell apart, not to mention our business partnership.

And on top of that, I had a huge amount of debt to repay because of that failed business down in Costa Rica.

So it was a stressful year. And really, I can't explain why I had to stop being a raw foodist overnight and start eating everything else in huge quantities, but what I *can* say is that I don't think I would have been able to go through that experience eating just fruits and vegetables. In fact, I'm quite confident I wouldn't have been able to do it.

The strangest thing is, I only gained weight toward the very end of that year.

Of course I was overeating. But my body was definitely using the food, and to be honest, I felt physically fine. Psychologically, the experience was very difficult, but I had all the energy I needed to get through it, which was the most important thing. From six months of "massive eating," I only gained about ten pounds. And then it only took me a couple months to lose it. At that point, I stopped overeating so much, and tried to find my balance again. I went back to being mostly raw and mostly vegan, but as with my initial dental health experiment, I was never the same. I had discovered that "the perfect diet" may not work in all circumstances. I also found out how hard it is for raw foodists to do anything other than go from one extreme to another!

I eat a plant-based diet, but I'm not a vegan.

There have been many times I have eaten *like* a vegan, but for the past ten years or so I've always consumed some animal products on some occasions. This has mostly been only occasional consumption, but sometimes I've eaten them on a regular basis.

The main reason I'm not a vegan is not because I particularly fear that my health will be worse if I abstain from animal products, or believe I "need" animal products. Rather, for me, the main reason is I enjoy having fewer restrictions in my diet, and I also think there's little evidence to show that a diet based on whole foods with lots of fruits and vegetables, with around 10% or fewer total calories coming from animal foods, is unhealthy. I do think that this small percentage of animal foods can only provide a more rounded nutritional plan overall; and no research, not even from the staunchest anti-meat advocates, has ever shown that consuming some animal protein in that amount is unhealthy.

Although my vegan identity died a long time ago, I feel great eating mostly plant-based meals, but like to have the option of eating some fish, meat and small amounts of dairy or eggs on occasion. Mostly, this gives me more options when traveling — which is something I enjoy — and the few times I eat out with friends or am invited at a friend or family member's house for dinner.

Has there ever been a vegan culture?

There's no major human culture in the world — anywhere — going back in time as long as you like — that has lived on a vegan diet. There are a few religious groups, such as Buddhists, that recommend a vegetarian diet, and many Buddhist monks are effectively vegan, since they avoid meat and live in parts of the word where dairy and eggs are seldom consumed. Big parts of India are vegetarian. The Jain religion of India has the strictest ban on animal product consumption of any religion. Based on the principle of doing no harm (*ahimsa*), it mandates avoidance not only of animal products but also of root vegetables, for fear of killing small bugs when harvesting them. However, the ambient Indian veneration of the cow means that dairy has never been completely banned within the religion, although abstention has been recommended—even more so by modern Jain leaders conscious of brutal dairy farm practices. Throughout the religion's history, many individual Jains have chosen to forego dairy in a strict interpretation of their religion's mandates. But there is no culture in the world that is *uniformly* vegan.

Only in the modern world do you find a vegan culture — one that is now spread across continents. But even then, most vegans do not stay pure vegans their whole lives.

According to a study published in Psychology Today, about 75% of vegetarians and vegans eventually return to meat or animal products. The average amount of time most people stay vegetarian is nine years.

I think the study matches my own experience of meeting many ex-vegetarians and ex-vegans over the years.

Ex-vegans and ex-vegetarians are now sharing their experiences on the Internet, upsetting current vegetarians and vegans. But ultimately, only a small percentage of people stay on a pure vegan diet for the rest of their lives, and almost never do you see generations after generations of people raised on a vegan diet.

About half of vegetarians give up meat for ethical reasons, just like I did, at the age of eighteen. The videos and pictures shared by animal activist groups of farm animals rolling in their own excrement all packed next to each other in "concentration camps" are disturbing enough to curb the appetite of the staunchest meat-eaters.

But many ex-vegetarians eventually discover they can buy grass-fed beef or other similar alternatives from farms near them, and change their ethically motivated diets accordingly.

Why has there been no vegan world culture?

Human cultures throughout the world have always eaten animal products — even cultures that were vegetarian for religious reasons. Buddhist monks sometimes receive fish as alms and accept it as providence.

Why is this?

There are several ways to answer the question. First of all, everywhere in the world, plant foods were only available seasonally in prehistoric times. The advent of agriculture set the scene for the starch-based (i.e. plant-based) diet, and storage methods quickly became sophisticated. But even with more plant food available year-round, and even if the proportion of meat in the diet decreased, animal products were still eaten. Animals that were a nuisance to the community were hunted. Beasts of burden or laying hens eventually reached the end of their working lives. Until very recently, humans have always lived with animals at very close quarters, and eating them has been part and parcel of that coexistence.

Another reason is nutritional. I won't be popular with the vegan community for bringing this up, but there are several important or even essential micronutrients that are either unobtainable from plant foods alone, or very difficult to obtain in the right form or quantity. I'm talking about Vitamins B12, D3, and K2; also the long chain omega-3 fatty acids DHA and EPA, and certain amino acids important for muscle building like carnitine and carnosine. Of course I'm not saying that our ancestors consciously ate animal products to ward off these deficiencies! Someone might turn the reasoning around and say that we can't obtain those nutrients from plant foods alone *because* we lived with animals and ate them and their products for so long.

Either way, it's food for thought.

Most of us no longer live at such close quarters with animals—or even with the plant foods that we eat, either. The plus side of this separation from the land is our great liberty to choose a career without having to set aside time to go plow the fields or harvest the nuts, all the while enjoying an unprecedented variety and quantity of foods *year round*. Would-be vegans and raw foodists have never had it better. But they should consider themselves pioneers or experimenters, and remember how unusual our modern food situation is in the historical context.

Ex-Vegans

The popularity of vegan diets has grown in the last decade, because the Internet enables vegans to connect with each other, exchange ideas, and also promote their lifestyle. At the same time, you can find many "ex-vegans" who passionately share how the vegan diet didn't work for them and why they're eating animal foods now.

These stories are particularly embarrassing for the vegan movement as a whole because they discourage many people from trying out a vegan diet, and encourage existing vegans who are experiencing problems to give up the diet too.

It's sometimes difficult to understand what is really going on because in many cases people are self-diagnosing their problems and coming up with their own explanations. Many ex-vegans don't just include a little meat back into their diet, but actually go to the opposite extreme, actually seeking out foods high in cholesterol, thinking that a diet very high in saturated animal fats is good for the body.

While I'm not negating someone's experience, many vegans are prone to excess, and they often seem to transform their zeal *for* veganism into zeal *against* veganism in their post-vegan anger. They go from believing that a vegan diet is the right diet for *everybody* to claiming that *nobody* can be healthy on a vegan diet. They go from thinking that a diet without any animal foods is best, to thinking that a diet with *lots* of animal foods is best. The truth is probably somewhere in between.

Often, these ex-vegans have little nutritional knowledge, and while they may be accurate in their perception that something is wrong with their health, their self-diagnosis is not complete, and their adjustments not clear. Many people add eggs back into their diet in order to get more protein, not realizing that a large egg only contains 6 grams of protein, less than a cup of soy milk.

Many people abandon vegan diets for various reasons, but the biggest one is because of health. They didn't feel well as vegans, so they quit. I personally struggled to find balance, coming from the idealism of the raw food diet, so it was important for me to eat a diet that wasn't overly restricted.

Can You Be Healthy on a Vegan Diet?

You can certainly be healthy and obtain all the nutrients you need to thrive on a vegan diet, but it requires more planning than to do so on a plant-based diet that includes *some* animal products. The reason is pretty simple: humans are not actually *vegan creatures*; therefore a vegan diet is not common in human societies. Eating a wider variety of foods —coming both from plant and animal sources (with plants predominating) makes it easier to get everything your body needs.

I will agree with the overwhelming scientific consensus that a plant-*based* diet is the healthiest diet. The vast majority of top scientists and longevity experts agree with this.

But the real question, one that even many plant-based advocates have been debating for quite a while, is whether a 100% plant-based diet is superior to an almost identical diet but with 5 to 10% of calories from clean animal sources.

In other words, we know that people get sick when they get most of their calories from animal sources. Too much is too much. However, are there some benefits to small amounts? Even well-known plant-based advocates such as T. Colin Campbell only found health problems in their studies when over 10% of total calories were consumed from animal sources. In *Eat To Live*, Dr. Joel Fuhrman also agrees with this conclusion (p.97) and incorporates it in his own recommendations—"No more than 10 percent of your total calories should come from animal foods" (p.164). On the other hand, Dr. John McDougall says that even if a small amount of animal foods is not unhealthy, any amount of animal products in the diet is still dangerous because the behaviors are too difficult to change, and it's too difficult to be moderate. Citing behavioral issues and taste addictions, he recommends keeping clear boundaries. (e.g. http://www. lanimuelrath.com/diet-nutrition/mcdougall-vs-fuhrman-notes-for-you-from-the-great-plant-based-doctors-debate/)

Animal Foods in the Diet by Percentage of Calories

Calories	5%	10%
2000 calorie diet	100 calories: 1 large egg OR, 2.5 ounces salmon, OR 6 ounces of whole milk yogurt	200 calories: 2 large eggs OR 5 ounces salmon, or 3.5 ounces filet mignon steak
3000 calorie diet	150 calories: 2 medium eggs OR 1 small filet of cod (5 ounces) OR	300 calories: 5 ounces of lamb, or 12 ounces red snapper, or 12 ounces skinless chicken breast

Recommended Supplements for Vegans and Raw Foodists

A few supplements are necessary on a vegan or raw vegan diet, although many of these supplements are also necessary on diets that contain animal foods.

B12

Unfortunately, some people in the raw food world give the bad advice to "wait until you have a deficiency" before supplementing with vitamin B12. Or they maintain that vitamin B12 can be obtained by consuming unwashed organic produce. B12 deficiency can cause irreversible neurological damage. Supplementation is a requirement for all vegans and for anyone with low levels of vitamin B12 (which becomes harder to assimilate the older you get).

Vitamin B12 tablets should be sublingual—to be held under the tongue for a couple of minutes, which is a fast track for absorption. Hold it under your tongue, chew it, or blend it with your food. Don't swallow it whole. Make sure to pick a supplement made with methylcobalamin and not the more common *cyanocobalamin*. Only 25 or so micrograms of methylcobalamin are necessary, but for the other kind, it could be as high as 2000 micrograms.

The recommended dose (for a methylcobalamin supplement) is 25 to 100 micrograms per day, or 1000 micrograms a few times a week. Start with at least 2000 micrograms for a few weeks. Get a blood test done, and if you are deficient, you might need higher doses, or injections.

Vitamin D

This is not a vegan issue, although some animal products, like fatty fish, have stored vitamin D. 1000 IUs of vitamin D daily is advisable, although this can vary greatly depending on the sun exposure where you live and how dark- or light-skinned you are. The D3 form of the vitamin is more absorbable.

Iodine

Raw foodists who avoid salt or vegans who only use sea salt are at risk for iodine deficiencies. Iodine can be found in food, but depleted soils means reduced levels in food too. Use a supplement providing about 100 micrograms a day, or use iodized salt instead of sea salt.

Calcium

You can get enough calcium from greens, but it can be difficult. If you don't consume at least four or five cups of cooked greens a day (or probably two to three times that amount raw), of a variety of greens like kale, then you may not be getting enough calcium. You could get enough if you make regular green smoothies and cook a bunch of greens every night. Otherwise, take a calcium supplement (ideally one containing vitamin D so you get both nutrients at the same time).

Keep in mind that some kinds of greens contain calcium, but because they also contain oxalic acid, most of the calcium is not absorbed. Besides spinach, beet greens and Swiss chards also have the same property. I suspect that baby spinach is more absorbable because it tastes less like oxalic acid, but I could be wrong. Further research is needed in this regard.

I know, I know, we've heard the story that the countries that have the highest calcium consumption also have the highest rates of osteoporosis. This is blamed on excess animal protein consumption, which causes calcium to leach out of the body or be used up to neutralize the acidity of such diets. Asian countries are known for relatively low calcium intake (although they do eat a lot of calcium-containing greens, such as bok choy, mustard greens, and others), and also have low rates of osteoporosis. The Vegan RD writes:

> ". . .with so many variables among different countries and cultures, it's hard to draw real conclusions. For example, Asians have a slightly different hip structure than other ethnic groups which makes it more resistant to fracture. That might explain why Asians have fewer hip fractures than Westerners but have similar rates of spinal fractures and also similar bone density.

> There are also geographic and cultural explanations for the differences in hip fracture rates. Falling is a big cause of hip fracture and for a number of reasons, Asians fall less often than Westerners. The comparison also doesn't control for physical activity, which is very protective of bone health, or for childbearing. Women in some of the countries in the comparisons have many more pregnancies than Westerners, and there is some evidence that pregnancy improves bone health (although not all studies agree about that)."

In the end, it doesn't matter where you get your calcium from, and dairy products are certainly not necessary in that regard. However, you have to make sure you get a good amount, close to the recommendation of 1000 mg a day. This is doable if you consume a LOT of greens; otherwise, take a calcium supplement.

Iron

Iron may or may not be a problem for some women. There's no standard recommendation for vegans, so ask your health professional.

DHA/EPA

I talked about this in my book *Raw Food Controversies*. Fish-eaters can get plenty of these long-chain fatty acids essential for brain health and reducing inflammation, but they *could* be lacking in vegan diets. The body can make DHA and EPA from other omega-3 fatty acids such as ALA found in flax and chia seeds especially, but the theory is that some people may not be able to make that conversion very well, so would need to get it from either fish or supplements.

A lack of DHA can cause or exacerbate depression, and produce other symptoms, such as fatigue.

Vegan DHA supplements, made from algae oil, are available.

Cooked Foods to Eat

Going from an *exclusion* to *inclusion* mindset requires you to think first about the foods you're going to eat, before listing all everything you should eliminate from your diet. Health is a lot about what you *don't* eat, but it's also about all of the healthy foods that you eat. And naturally, as long as you're eating healthy food there's little space left for unhealthy foods.

We've already covered some essential raw food habits you should hold on to. Once you've determined which of those habits are the most important for you to implement, and *when* you're going to implement them, then you can think about the cooked foods you're going to eat in addition to the raw foods. Those healthy cooked foods will naturally replace the other foods you've been eating in the past, or would be tempted to eat.

There's nothing revolutionary here. Healthy cooked foods will usually meet all these criteria:

- **Whole foods** — Grains will have the fiber intact, and will not be processed into flours. Fats will come from whole foods (nuts, seeds, etc.) rather than oils, but if oils are consumed, they will be of the highest quality, and usually added after cooking.

- **Cooking method** — Cooking in water (boiling or steaming) will be preferred to high-temperature cooking like baking. Frying will be avoided, but stir-frying in almost no oil will be accepted. Barbecuing meats will be avoided, and if meats are consumed grilled, they will be marinated first in a marinade containing acids (like lime juice). Good quality meats can be consumed rare, and a lot of fish can be consumed raw or rare.[9]

- **Types of food** — Foods from the fruit and vegetable kingdom

---

9   Needless to say, precautions should be taken when eating raw or rare animal products. Certain types of fish, like wild salmon, should never be eaten raw—see this article for the graphic details! http://www.gourmet.com/foodpolitics/2008/08/raw-salmon-tapeworm.

(including all root vegetables and squash) will be preferred to an abundance of grain products. Beans can always be enjoyed. If animal foods are consumed, they are a supplement to a plant-based diet and not the main source of calories or fat.

- **Source** — Fruits and vegetables are healthy whether conventionally grown or organic, although you may want to check out the Environmental Working Group's "Dirty Dozen" most contaminated produce items, which you may prefer to buy organic, and "Clean Fifteen" fruits and vegetables with the lowest pesticide residues, which you can probably buy conventional without lying awake at night http://www.ewg.org/foodnews/. But special care must be taken when sourcing animal products, which tend to be more contaminated with pesticide residues from the plant food the animal eats, which concentrate in the animal's tissues, as well as growth hormones and antibiotics. So is it important to source organic animal products? Yes, I believe it is. Always remember that YOU are what the animals you eat were. In other words, whatever the animals ingest, you ingest as well when you eat animal products. Organic dairy farmers and ranchers use pure water, quality feed, and provide healthy pastures and fresh air for their animals. This ensures their organically raised animals grow at their natural pace, without artificial growth hormones. The "use of antibiotics, synthetic hormones, and genetically modified organisms to intensify production in conventional agriculture practices, which give rise to serious health questions," are excluded from their operations. Additionally, going back to our discussion of omega 6 and omega 3 fats, if you eat commercial animal products from big factory farms you will not be getting enough omega 3 fatty acids and other important nutrients. If you consume animal products, the best sources of omega 3 will be from wild, fresh-caught fish like salmon, tuna, and halibut, and from free-range eggs and organic grass-fed beef.

Some unnecessary concerns

People often get obsessed about small details that don't really matter that much. It's much better to focus your energy on the 20% of things that will give you 80 or 90% of your results, rather than wasting your precious time on minutiae or perfectionism. Often, certain obsessions or fears entertained by the natural health community are based more on conspiracy theories than real science.

Avoiding GMO's

Okay, I might not be very popular for saying this, but I personally don't think we should absolutely fear genetically modified foods. This goes against the fear campaign that almost everyone involved in natural health has been spreading. I think there are two sides to every issue, and it's really important not to blindly accept something as *truth*. Some people blindly accept what the media tells them. Others see everything as a conspiracy theory. Generally, raw foodists belong to the latter category. GMOs are a tricky issue involving much more than health, including farmer's rights, plant gene "trademarks," and more. But ultimately, it's a technology that is necessary to feed a growing population, and we won't be able to avoid it completely. After having looked seriously at both sides of the issue, I do not think there's a reason to be afraid of it either. We can be concerned, but not reject it completely. In my opinion, fruits and vegetables that have been somewhat genetically modified and already on the market, such as Hawaiian papayas, are perfectly healthy and safe to eat, and I personally make absolutely no efforts to avoid them. A good book to read, written by an organic farmer, that looks at this important issue in a balanced way, is *Tomorrow's Table* (by Pamela C. Ronald and R. W. Adamchak). I recommend checking it out if you're serious about understanding this issue.

Eating only local foods

Being a *locavore* may be trendy but it's not necessarily rational. The fact is that transportation only represents a tiny part of the carbon footprint of food, and in fact driving to go buy your fruit produces more CO_2 than those foods being efficiently transported by boat or plane halfway across the world. Studies have shown that purchasing local foods that have been refrigerated long-term (such as apples) is worse for the environment than purchasing out-of-season imported foods from faraway countries like New Zealand. I think the *locavore* trend is just another Western obsession with doing everything that *goes against the man*, as a sort of statement against an illusory oppressor, loosely defined as *globalism*. The truth is that globalism is one of the greatest steps that humankind has ever taken. In fact, the entire raw food movement would never have occurred without global trade systems that allow almost anyone, anywhere in the world, to eat a variety of foods previously unavailable to entire generations.

Obsession with food combining

There is some truth to the efficacy of food combining, in the sense that simplifying one's eating pattern is generally a healthier thing to do and will lead to more optimal digestion. However, food combining rules are not based on sound science. I've noticed that it's not so much about the *combination* but rather the amount. If I eat several ounces of nuts along with several ounces of dried fruit, I invariably get gas and a mild form of indigestion. But if I eat just one ounce of nuts with a handful of dried fruit, I'm fine.

The Healthiest Cooked Foods

Cooked foods that meet the criteria for healthy food can be included in your Beyond Raw plan, in the context of everything we've discussed. Although there are no true "superfoods," there are certain cooked foods that have certain benefits and should be included more often in our diets. Let's take a look.

Sweet potatoes

I've had a thing for sweet potatoes lately. During WW2, the Japanese living on the island of Okinawa lived on a diet composed almost exclusively of sweet potatoes. The Asian variety of sweet potato is blue inside, not orange. But the vegetable is very simple. Is it a coincidence that these people ended up being the longest-lived people in the world?

No doubt, a diet composed mostly of sweet potatoes with a few other things would be Spartan. But it can also give the body everything it needs. Compared to other complex carbs, sweet potatoes contain more vitamins, especially beta-carotene.

Most people who are sensitive to carbs handle sweet potatoes very well. Baking them is common, but I prefer to peel them, slice them about an inch thick, and steam them in a pot with just enough water to last through the cooking process. I don't cook them until they are mushy. I leave a little crunch to them.

Cooked that way, they'll keep a few days in the fridge. That way, you can enjoy sweet potatoes often without having to worry about baking them for an hour.

Winter Squash

This is a type of food most people didn't grow up eating in North America, but they're true superfoods. Again, they're alkaline-forming and super-rich in minerals, and they fill you up like potatoes or bread, but they're much easier to digest, and surprisingly low in calories.

Butternut squash is a classic, but my favorite is the red kuri squash called "potimarron" in French. The texture of this one is truly creamy and delicious, and you can cook it with the skin on.

Beans

According to the book *The Blue Zones*, one thing that all long-lived people in the world have in common is that they eat beans.

Black beans, soy beans, chickpeas, lentils…. beans are a slow-digesting carb that will give you sustained energy. It's generally the food that "junkfood vegans" don't eat enough of.

My favorite beans are black beans, popular in Latin America. I cook them for about two hours without soaking (but with a quick rinse), with bay leaves, garlic, and one small peeled potato (which I throw away after cooking).

Steamed Greens

Greens are healthy in all their forms, but the advantage of slightly steaming them is that they become much easier to chew, digest and assimilate. Blending or juicing them also achieves similar purposes.

Certain greens are just not that enjoyable to eat raw, like chard and kale. I know, I know, there are little tricks to make them more "chewable" but it's often not worth it because cooking them for a few minutes does not really alter their nutritional value and makes them so much easier to eat.

I like to steam kale and add it to salads that are otherwise raw, along with a creamy dressing.

Mushrooms

Only Americans add raw mushrooms to salad. This practice is deemed very strange by Europeans, who always cook mushrooms.

There's a reason to cook mushrooms. Their cell walls are extremely difficult to digest. So if you eat raw mushrooms, you just don't benefit from them. Cooking them releases significantly more nutritional value. It also destroys some compounds that could make them irritating or toxic in the raw state.

But why eat mushrooms then?

New research shows that they contain powerful compounds that can prevent and fight cancer. That's why Dr. Fuhrman, author of *Eat to Live*, so enthusiastically recommends them.

They also fill you up without containing many calories. Plus, they can be delicious too!

Rice

The fear campaign against carbs, and especially rice, is largely undeserved. Rice is a staple for billions of people who have remained lean, active and healthy eating it for hundreds of generations.

Rice is generally well tolerated by most people who are sensitive to other grains, or can't handle gluten.

Brown rice is considered the healthiest, but its phytate contain may make the minerals less accessible. Nonetheless, it's rich in fiber and easy to digest, and won't make anybody fat anytime soon. It's almost impossible to gain weight on a brown rice-based diet because it's just so filling with so few calories.

White rice, although often categorized as "junk food," is actually a very neutral food that is so easy to digest that it can often be used by people who need extra energy and are sensitive to other types of complex carbs.

But don't rule out other types of rice. There's about 9 types of rice that I personally use and rotate.

Red rice, Black Rice — I love these unusual rices which are rich in antioxidants. Available in Asian markets or health food stores.

Jasmine rice, Basmati — Best to serve with curry and very aromatic!

Parboiled rice. This rice has been partially boiled with the husk and bran to incorporate some of the bran's nutrients into the interior of the rice. So, it's white rice with a nutritional profile similar to brown rice. It's often used in Caribbean rice and beans, and is quick to cook.

Sweet rice (or "sticky" rice) – Often used in making Asian dessert recipes, such as sticky rice with mangoes and coconut milk.

Let's not even get into the other varieties of rice used to making sushi rice, risotto, etc.!

Cooked Tomato Products

Both raw and cooked tomatoes are healthy. I don't subscribe to always trying to isolate specific nutrients in food, such as lycopene in tomatoes. But the fact is that certain nutrients are easier to assimilate in cooked foods, while others that are too sensitive to heat should be obtained from raw foods.

Raw tomatoes are excellent, but cooked tomatoes can make life worth living sometimes. I'm talking about the incredible aroma of home-made tomato sauce. And it's true that cooking tomatoes boosts their antioxidant content.

About... Fat

Health theories come and go. Some are valid, some are not. Some are valid in certain contexts, but useless in others.

For many years, my hobbyhorse in the raw food movement was fat versus fruit. Many years ago, I came to the realization that the main reasons people were failing so miserably on the raw food diet were because:

- They didn't consume enough calories
- The calories they consumed mostly came from fat (in some cases 60%+)
- They failed to get enough carbohydrates
- In the context of a high sugar diet (from fruit), the fat content of their diet created a horrible combination, causing blood sugar imbalances, yeast infections, and other problems

There's no doubt that on a 100% raw food diet, fat can be either your friend or your enemy. The biggest problem with a raw vegan diet is that calories can only come from two sources:

- Fat (avocados, nuts, seeds, etc.)
- Sugar (from fruit)

Complex carbohydrates are not allowed, and when they are eaten raw, the starch in them is not digested. Protein sources are also typically verboten —on a raw food diet concentrated protein sources could only come from animal products.

The problem is that raw fat sources are not healthy in large quantities. Getting most of one's calories from nuts and seeds means creating a huge omega 6 to omega 3 imbalance in the body. Nuts contain mostly omega 6 polyunsaturated fats, and the ratio to omega 3s is often very skewed.

Some omega 6 fatty acids are essential; they are necessary for human health but the body can't synthesize them. You have to get them through food. Along with omega 3 fatty acids, omega 6 fatty acids play a crucial role in brain function, as well as normal growth and development. Also known as polyunsaturated fatty acids (PUFAs), they help stimulate skin and hair growth, maintain bone health, regulate metabolism, and maintain the reproductive system.

However, a *healthy diet* contains a balance of omega-3 and omega-6 fatty acids. Omega 3s are anti-inflammatory and make cell walls softer and more permeable. Omega 6s ensure the cell walls are not too soft, but when not balanced by adequate omega 3s, they are pro-inflammatory and can promote cardiovascular disease, cancer, and inflammatory and autoimmune disease in general. Omega-3 fat deficiencies can lead to increased inflammation in your body, which predisposes you to chronic diseases like diabetes, allergies, and problems with mood and memory.

Both the absolute quantity of omega 6 and the ratio between omega 6 and 3 are important. The typical American diet tends to contain 14-25 times more omega 6 fatty acids than omega 3 fatty acids. The ideal ratio is thought to be 3:1 or 4:1 omega 6 to omega 3; the ratio in hemp seeds and walnuts, for example, but some believe the ratio should be closer to 1:1. Flax and chia seeds contain significantly more omega 3 than omega 6, which means they can be used "remedially" to balance out the results of nut and seed consumption.

The Mediterranean diet has a healthier balance between omega 3 and omega 6 fatty acids. Many studies have shown that people who follow this diet are less likely to develop heart disease. The Mediterranean diet does not include much meat from omnivores like pigs and chickens (high in omega 6 fatty acids); meat from herbivores allowed to eat grass rather than grain has a better ratio and lamb is popular in the Mediterranean. Although grains have a high omega 6 to 3 ratio, their consumption in the Mediterranean diet is balanced by fresh fruits and vegetables, fish, olive oil, and garlic, which are higher in omega 3.

The types of omega 3 and omega 6 fats you consume matter as much as the ratio. All dietary fats should come from whole foods that are organic, unprocessed and unrefined. Oils/fats you should avoid include corn, canola, cottonseed, and soy oils, and margarine.

There are also problems with too much fat in the diet, even if it comes mostly from monounsaturated sources like avocados or olives. First of all, it's incredibly boring. Avocados and oils are also quite heavy if they can't be "diluted" with complex carbohydrates. And a high-fat diet makes the blood sluggish, decreases insulin sensitivity and, without enough carbohydrates, will not provide a feeling of energy.

When you add a lot of sugar (from fruit) on top of that, you have a recipe for disaster. Large quantities of sugar from fruit in the context of a diet extremely rich in omega 6 polyunsaturated fat, and just lots of fat in general, can led to extreme health issues, such as:

- Inflammation throughout the body
- Blood sugar swings
- Elevated blood sugar, even leading to diabetes
- Frequent fungal infections (including candida)

For these reasons, I previously recommended limiting fat to 15% of total calories, or less. For a while, I was following the lead of Dr. Doug Graham, who recommends less than 10%. But in practice, I found that 10% of calories from fat was too low for most people, and led to other problems, including:

- Dry and aged-looking skin
- Dry and raggedy hair
- Hormonal problems in some people, leading to hair loss in women and lack of libido in men

In the last few years, I've been experimenting with the fat percentage in my diet. I went below 10% for many periods, and tried other amounts as well.

I discovered that in the context of a 100% raw food diet, and I would say even an 80% or 90% raw food diet, where *most* of the calories are coming from fruit, between 12 and 17% fat in the diet is probably ideal. The actual percentage depends on a lot of factors, and I think it's best for most people to experiment to see what works best for them.

At the moment I do not eat an 80 or 90% raw diet. I'm probably more like 50% raw. But as I said elsewhere, I don't actually calculate the percentages anymore. It's more the percentage of your diet that comes from fruits, vegetables, nuts, and seeds that counts — whether those foods are raw or not.

I discovered that in the context of my current diet, I can increase the fat content and not get the problems I would otherwise expect if my diet were high in fruit sugar. In other words, restricting the fat content to 10 or 15% of total calories seems more important on a fruit-based diet, but less so on a more varied diet.

I would probably still be eating 10 to 15% fat if I hadn't started to notice something I didn't like. I found my skin was often very dry. Especially my forehead, where my skin would flake daily. My hands also started to get dry. I used moisturizers to take care of the problem. But then, another thing started to bother me. I noticed that over the last few years, my hair started to take on a sort of "raggedy" look. It was very dry, and I couldn't fix the problem by using conditioners. It's not just that it was dry. It seemed to have lost its *shine* and just looked dead and unhealthy. And I noticed the same in many other vegans following a low-fat diet.

At that time, I was probably eating 10 to 18% fat in my diet. My average was probably closer to 14-15% in practice. So as an experiment, I started to increase the fat percentage in my diet. The main change I made was to allow myself to eat some olive oil — maybe a tablespoon a day. I also started to eat nuts more regularly, and avocados made a more frequent appearance on my menu.

I started to lose my fear of fat. I ate an ounce of nuts as a snack every day. I dropped a half up to a whole avocado on my salad, and I ate some fatty fish like wild salmon a couple times a week.

Within about a month, I noticed a huge difference in my skin. Even in the dead of winter, my skin was no longer flaky. But the biggest difference was my hair. It finally felt alive again, and was not so dry-looking. It felt great to the touch, even without much conditioner.

Now, some people who promote a very low-fat diet will say my skin just got greasy. But I felt the amount of oil produced by my skin was just right, enough to protect it from the elements. Overly dry skin, on the other hand, didn't seem right to me.

So at the moment I probably get around 18-25% of my calories from fat. This is something I could never have done on an all-raw diet because too much fat, combined with lots of fruit sugar, would have caused many problems. But all the problems caused by fat only seem to occur on a very high-fat diet, and when the diet is also high in sugar (natural or otherwise).

So for raw food diets, I still recommend keeping the fat percentage fairly low; 15% or less.

Saturated Fat

The status of saturated fats, found in butter and land animals, but also in tropical nuts like coconut, pili nut and palm fruit, is less cut and dried than it used to be in the health food world. This is mostly because the relationship between saturated fat and cholesterol, on the one hand, and heart disease on the other, has been called into serious question. Meanwhile, important benefits of foods containing this fat have been shown. I'm going to leave aside the other foods for now and focus on coconut, as that's what's most applicable for my readers.

First off, just like there are different polyunsaturated fatty acids, there are over twenty different kinds of saturated fat. Coconut fat contains around 30% medium chain triglycerides (MCTs), known to have metabolic-boosting properties. Some of these fatty acids, lauric and caprylic acids, have antifungal action, and are also present in human breast milk. Because it contains almost no polyunsaturated fat, coconut does not contribute to the omega 6 to 3 ratio imbalances.

Mature coconut meat, whether from a fresh brown coconut or the dried shredded coconut, is also very high in fiber. Between the fiber and the fat, this makes coconut a very filling food.

Some raw foodists went a little crazy with this information about the fats and told everyone coconut oil digests more like a carb than a fat, isn't really a fat, that it speeds up your metabolism so much that the more you eat of it the more weight you'll lose, etc., and all of a sudden somewhere in the mid-2000's, everyone was making raw desserts with about a quarter cup of coconut oil per serving, to firm up the already very heavy cashew-based cream mixed with agave. Try that in your belly for an afternoon! Do you think anyone lost weight from that?

Coconut oil is still oil, is still just as refined as a refined sugar, and I still don't recommend it.

However, between its high fiber content and the good qualities of its fat, mature coconut is a good food. The high fiber content almost ensures you won't eat too much—it's so filling, and your mouth will start to hurt if you are chewing it for too long. Coconut butter is different than coconut oil. It is like almond butter instead of almond oil: it contains the whole meat, but ground until the oils release and the fibers are mostly crushed. Like almond butter, it still retains a trace of the fibrous character. It can be mixed with water and used instead of coconut milk in curries.

Young coconut meat is another different source of coconut fat. Taken from immature "green" coconuts, which contain much more of the beloved coconut water, the meat is anything from a translucent gel to something firmer and harder, closer to mature coconut meat, depending on the level of maturity. This coconut meat is almost closer to avocado, and is gentle and easy to digest. There is much less fat in this stage of coconut meat, and almost no fiber. Instead, there is more simple sugar, giving it a subtly sweet taste. So young coconut is one of the unusual foods, also including the tropical fruit durian, that contains high amounts both of fat and sugar. Perhaps this explains why both are so popular among raw foodists.

Depending on where you live, young coconuts (generally sold with the husk shaved off so they are cut into white spheres with a pyramid shape at the top) can be hard-to-impossible to find, extremely expensive, and very hit-or-miss in terms of whether the water and meat inside are even any good when you get them open. On the other hand, in urban areas on the east and west coasts, you might be able to get them by the case in Chinatown districts, or even to buy the meat already removed from the coconut and fresh-packed in the water at natural food stores. Asian markets sometimes carry young coconut meat in the freezer section, but this often contains added sugar.

What Does Frederic Think About... Alcohol and Wine?

Drinking good wine, with good friends, eating good food, is the ultimate culinary experience for me, and one that helps me totally relax and not obsess so much about food for once.

What is the role of alcohol in the *Raw Freedom* program?

It's up to you. The truth is that wine, for example, is not totally good or totally bad for health. It's a question of context, personal sensitivity, and what it brings you as ROI.

Let's be honest. Wine is not a *health* product per se. However, you can incorporate some alcohol into an overall healthy lifestyle and get many benefits, both social and, to some degree, health-related.

Being able to drink *some* wine makes me *really* happy. Especially when I can share it with my friends. So the ROI of being able to drink wine is huge, and the negatives, with moderate consumption, are pretty low for me.

You've probably heard the theory that moderate alcohol consumption is good for health. Although a few studies once in a while contradict that claim, the vast majority of studies have found that a little wine or even beer is not likely to hurt you, and can even offer some benefits.

Often, health authorities come out with blanket recommendations that are supposed to apply to everybody. They will say, for example, that one drink a day and a maximum of ten a week (or less) is optimal for women, or two drinks a day or a maximum of fifteen a week is optimal for men. A drink is five ounces of wine, or twelve ounces of beer. However, the problem with such generic recommendations is that everybody is different.

For example, the same health authorities will say that up to 300 mg. of caffeine daily is perfectly acceptable for most people. Maybe, but I know in my case, I'm extremely sensitive to caffeine. Even 150 mg. of caffeine a day turns me into a depressed, irritable nut ball after just a few days.

On the other hand, alcohol doesn't affect me that much. For an experiment, I purchased a police-grade alcohol meter that measures the level of alcohol in the blood. It's mainly used by people who want to avoid DUI offenses after a night of partying.

One night, we shared some bottles of really good wine with a few friends for my brother's 30th birthday. At the end of the evening, everybody had drunk almost the exact same amount of wine. I made sure of that because I told everybody about the experiment. After five hours, we had each consumed about four glasses of wine.

My brother and I tested fairly similar. We were pretty much under 0.025 in blood alcohol level. My brother showed a higher resistance, being taller than me.

But one of our friends, who's about 20 years older, smaller, and of Haitian origin, registered at almost 0.08 in the test. This is actually over the legal limit for driving! But he'd had the same amount of wine! Obviously, his body was not processing alcohol as efficiently as my brother's and mine.

I don't routinely consume four glasses of wine. This was a party, and a fun one, but also an experiment. But now I don't even want to know how much alcohol it would take to send me over the legal limit!

The moral of the story is that everyone is different. If you decide to drink alcohol, then you should be aware of how your body reacts to it. For some people, the optimal amount of alcohol is zero. For others, it may be a glass of wine a couple times a week. Others can have more.

In the end, you should only choose to drink if it brings you a lot of benefits and few negatives.

In the scientific literature, benefits of moderate drinking that have been shown are:

- Reduced stress (for a big surprise!)
- Increased longevity as a result of reduced stress and better sleep
- Fewer heart attacks and strokes
- Less hypertension
- Less likely to develop Type 2 Diabetes
- Increases good (HDL) and lowers bad (LDL) cholesterol

However, there's no doubt that alcohol is a drug. Drugs generally have different effects, some that people view as beneficial, and some that could be detrimental. We already know the detrimental/addictive qualities of alcohol. As far as long-term health is concerned, it seems that a little alcohol is actually good for you, so long as these positives are not outweighed by negative effects for you personally.

My own view on alcohol is that if it helps your overall quality of life, enjoy some. If it doesn't, or you can't control yourself, or your body reacts extremely negatively, then avoid it. It's pretty simple.

But the truth is, the main benefit of alcohol is the reason it's been used in societies for thousands and thousands of years. Alcohol is a great social "glue" that can help people have a good time.

When people meet to share a festive meal, they open a bottle of wine and the conversation flows. People feel the relaxing effects of alcohol, they loosen up, leave their worries behind, and tongues loosen. When consumed in that context, a little wine or even beer can be extremely therapeutic on a psychological level.

If you don't already enjoy it there's no need to start, but if you're someone who likes a glass of light and fruity Pinot Noir on a Thursday night with your husband, or a glass of Syrah or micro-brewery porter with some friends, then by all means continue to do so.

I am not trying to convince you alcohol is healthy or that you need to have a glass of wine a day for heart health. Health is a complex subject and involves your entire lifestyle: stress levels, sense of pride and social belonging, fitness, etc. I don't find benefits to drinking wine every day myself.

The reason I enjoy drinking occasionally is the whole experience. I do enjoy spending time with friends and having a glass of good wine. I do enjoy the taste and complexities of wine. I also like how drinking a glass of wine along with a meal with friends makes me eat much slower than usual, and turns something that would be "just a meal" into a complete experience.

This is how I see it, and you're free to see it any other way. You're free to disagree with me, but I think you should also understand my point of view. A big part of my life was centered on "the raw food diet" in all forms, and a big part of my day was centered on food and food restrictions. At some point in my life, I was ready to move on and, while maintaining a super-healthy lifestyle, I wanted to be part of the social world — without this being a raw food potluck or other "raw-related" event.

During my raw food days, I did consume alcohol on occasion, such as a glass of wine, but for the most part I abstained. Nowadays, I have a simple rule that works for me. I call it the "Three Essential Elements of Drinking."

If I'm going to drink some alcohol, I want these three elements to be present:

- **Wine** — Although I do enjoy beer, I prefer good wine and the complexities and harmonies it can create with food.
- **Food** — Drinking a glass of wine with good food makes me enjoy my meal even more and helps me take my time eating it.
- **Friends** — In other words, no drinking alone.

With this simple rule, I have found I can incorporate a little wine-drinking into my life in what I consider a very healthy and rewarding way.

My philosophy will not work for everybody. I encourage you to think for yourself and decide where you stand on this matter, considering your health, how you react to alcohol, and if you see any positive benefits in it.

Various Diet Recommendations

This book is not aimed at covering all the food choices you *shouldn't* be making. There's plenty of information already available on the dangers of trans fat, fried foods, etc. Let's instead take a look at some basic diet recommendations. How you individualize the ratios is where it will all come together.

Eat a salad every day

The daily salad is important for a couple of reasons. First, we need to eat raw vegetables for all their nutrients, but we also need them for bulk. The big salad is one of those meals that gives you the "illusion" of being full without ingesting a lot of calories. In a raw food diet, that can be a problem. But in our case, because we're going to be eating other cooked foods for calories, we actually have to be more diligent in eating the daily salad because we don't want to overdo it with cooked starches and gain weight. Whether you eat your daily bowl of salad for breakfast, lunch or dinner doesn't really matter. Most people prefer to have it with their dinner meal. The bowl should be BIG. And try to put in a lot of vegetables, and a *variety* of vegetables. Don't be afraid of putting fruits too: kiwis, apples, pears, mangoes, and other fruits go well with salad meals. Legumes can be added to salad if you're going to make a meal out of it, and the dressing can be simple. My typical salad includes five to ten vegetables (lettuce, tomatoes, grated carrots, grated cabbage, etc.), one type of fruit (like a diced apple or pear), ½ cup to 1 cup of cooked legumes (like lentils), 1/3 to ½ an avocado OR 1 to 2 TBS of liquid tahini (the kind you buy at middle-eastern shops, not the health food store kind). To that I add a little bit of low-fat dressing, or simply some balsamic vinegar and a touch of salt, and I have a delicious salad!

Have a Green Smoothie, Green Juice, or other form of "Concentrated Greens"

Eating enough greens is important, and while the salad is great, you can often pack more greens into a green smoothie or "Savory Veggie Stew" than you could in an actual salad. You can also eat it much faster.

So I recommend a green smoothie every day, in addition to, or instead of, the daily salad. There are lots of books about green smoothies where you can find good recipes. I generally start with some water or almond milk. (Keep in mind that I need more calories that you probably do, so make sure to adapt it to your needs.) Then I throw in a few ripe bananas, and one other kind of fruit (like mango, berries, etc). I blend the whole thing, and only after blending, pack in as many greens as I can. I will usually go through half a large container of baby spinach, or an entire romaine lettuce (not a big one).

An alternative to the green smoothie is the Savory Veggie Stew, a delicious dinner meal developed by my friend Roger Haeske. It's even healthier than the green smoothie. Find out more at **www.veggiestews. com**

Eat cooked greens

This is something I'm not really doing on a regular basis, but I'm trying to incorporate. Greens are so good for you that there's a good chance you're not eating enough of them, even if you have a daily salad and green smoothie. The advantage of cooking greens is that they pack down to a very manageable size, and tougher greens, like kale, are much easier to digest after a few minutes of steaming.

One idea is to always include greens when you cook soups. Another is to buy a lot of kale and cook it ahead of time. Cooked kale will keep a couple of days (but not much longer) in the fridge, and it's a great addition to salads.

Eat fruit

I could have talked about fruit first, but eating fruit is too easy. The amount of fruit in your diet should be influenced by your activity level, and also the amount of other (cooked) carbs you eat. The more cooked carbs you eat, the less fruit you will need. Your body only needs so many calories and carbs, so if you eat a lot of rice and beans, you won't be craving as much fruit.

On a 100% raw food diet, getting enough calories from fruit can be a huge problem. However, on a diet that incorporates cooked foods, in some cases you may have to *limit* fruit if you're not planning on reducing caloric intake from other categories.

Eat as much fruit as you need to feel satisfied. But if you've been living on a fruit-based diet and you *want* to transition away, it's advisable to temporarily limit your fruit consumption to three to four pieces a day. The reason is that a fruitarian, or even a low-fat 100% raw foodist, has trained their body to use fruit as a main source of calories. So when they start eating other foods, they'll usually overeat by eating a similar quantity of fruit, and then adding cooked foods on top of it. You want to train your body to utilize other categories of food. Plus, you've been eating enough fruit to feed a small army, so taking a break won't hurt. It's all about training your body to digest other foods, so if you need to, take a break from fruit. You'll be happy to come back to it later.

I personally cannot think of a fruit that I don't enjoy. Fruits are best eaten whole and not blended, unless you do it in green smoothies.

Eat nuts

Many raw foodists overdo it on nuts, and end up with some serious health problems. It may sound crazy, but I know people who ate an entire jar of almond butter every day! I certainly could polish off half a jar myself back in the day...

Now the fact that nuts can be overdone on a raw food diet doesn't mean they're not healthy. They're extremely nutrient dense; it's just that they're also extremely calorie dense, so a little goes a long way. Nuts and seeds contain high-quality protein in varying amounts, from macadamia nuts, which contain almost no protein at all, to hemp seeds, which are 50% protein and contain all the essential amino acids.

With the exception of hemp, flax, and chia seeds, and walnuts, nuts and seeds have far more than the optimal 4:1 omega 6 to omega 3 ratio—*thousands* to one in the case of nuts like almonds, Brazil nuts, peanuts and sunflower seeds. However, nuts are also very high in vitamin E, a potent antioxidant that protects this unstable fat from oxidation. Aside from walnuts, nuts and seeds also have far more of their fat as monounsaturated fat with smaller amounts of the omega polyunsaturated fats, so despite the bad ratios, they shouldn't be a problem when consumed in moderation.

Nuts are high in B vitamins (not including B12). They are high in fiber and in minerals. Pumpkin seeds are famously high in zinc, essential for metabolism and hormonal functions. One single Brazil nut will give you your total daily requirement of selenium, a trace mineral crucial for thyroid health that can otherwise be hard to get.

Epidemiological evidence is mounting that people who eat nuts are less likely to develop heart disease and gallstones. Women who eat nuts have also been shown to be less likely to develop diabetes. There's also some evidence that nut-eaters have reduced incidence of high blood pressure, cancer, and inflammation. In interventional studies, despite their fatty nature, nuts consistently *lower* cholesterol. They also have a positive impact on belly fat (the dangerous kind), and metabolic syndrome.

Finally, both epidemiological studies and clinical trials consistently show that nuts help *prevent* obesity; that they may even help in weight loss![10]

---

10   A good source for this data is "Health Benefits of Nut Consumption" by Emilio Ros
     http://www.ncbi.nlm.nih.gov/pmc/articles/PMC3257681/

Now, this conclusion wasn't reached by examining people eating raw burgers made from a pound of walnuts and sunflower seeds, or raw cheesecakes with a half cup of cashews and a quarter cup of coconut oil in a single agave-sweetened slice. Just saying.

The right amount of nuts for most people to eat daily is one ounce. If you're more active, have two ounces a day. If you eat your nuts as a snack and chew them well, you'll see how satisfying they can be.

All the research that's been done on nuts and health show they are beneficial. But I know you can be afraid of nuts when you're coming from a raw food background. I certainly was sick of nuts for many years after having relied on them so much in my early raw food days.

Now, I enjoy a daily ounce of nuts, chewed well, usually as an afternoon snack or with breakfast.

Almonds are my favorite. But other nuts are great too. Walnuts are excellent for health.

If you're trying to lose weight, eat some almonds. Recent research demonstrated that people eating almonds daily lost more weight than those on a low-fat diet with the same number of calories. Participants in the study saw a reduction of 18% in body weight, compared to only 11% in the non-almond group. And remember, both groups ate the same number of calories. The almond-eaters saw their blood pressure drop by 11%, compared to no change in the non-almond group. Other improvements were noticed in cholesterol levels. Besides being good for you and full of nutrients, almonds have very tough fiber that acts as a physical barrier to fat. So one reason they can help you lose weight is that you feel full eating them, but the body is not able to absorb all the calories. (Source: **http://www.webmd.com/diet/news/20031107/almonds-may-help-in-weight-loss**)

As a raw foodist, I got into nut butters because they are great for dressings. But lately I've been enjoying *chewing* on nuts, and find them extremely satisfying that way, especially if you truly take the necessary time and effort to chew them properly. I use tahini in salads sometimes, but I prefer to eat other nuts whole.

Eat beans every day

Raw foodists and natural hygienists claim that cooked mature legumes are unhealthy. Arguments used are the same old "this is not a food you would find in nature," and the usual raw food BS.

But the proof is in the results.

In 2005, National Geographic magazine commissioned a study on the "Blue Zones," which are places in the world where longevity is *currently* exceptionally long, and also verifiable. We are not talking about the Hunzas or the Vilcabambas, tribes renowned for longevity but with no verifiable records to prove it. The researchers wanted to locate the current hot spots for longevity, where they could interview real centenarians and ask them what they did.

One of the researchers, Dan Buettner, wrote a book titled *The Blue Zones: Lessons For Living Longer From the People Who've Lived the Longest* detailing the findings and offering some suggestions that anyone might follow based on commonalities between the diverse places.

The five identified regions were:

Sardinia, Italy — there's a "hot spot" in the mountain villages, where men reach the age of 100 with amazing frequency.

The island of Okinawa, Japan —has long been reputed to have the most centenarians on earth.

Loma Linda, California — where a religious group, the Seventh-Day Adventists, rank among the longest-lived people in America, and the world.

The Nicoya Peninsula in Costa Rica – not all of Costa Rica is reputed for longevity, but the inhabitants of this part of the country are.

Ikaria, Greece – a unique island whose inhabitants have the highest odds of reaching the age of 90.

What's interesting about the Blue Zones is that all these different cultures were doing different things. But one thing that *all* cultures had in common, from the Costa Ricans of the Nicoya Peninsula to the Ikarian islanders, was *the regular consumption of beans and legumes!* Along with a few other factors (strong family bonds, no smoking, a plant-based diet, physical activity), bean consumption was among the few things ALL cultures had in common.

So to anyone who would claim that beans are not healthy, I would reply that all of the longest-lived cultures eat them. Beat that!

Whole beans is the one category of food many vegans don't consume enough of. In the Beyond Raw program, beans are very important. Most people should be eating about one cup of cooked beans every day.

Limit refined oils

As explained previously, oils can be a problem because they are a concentrated source of calories. So if you're trying to lose weight, you should limit or eliminate oils and favor whole-food sources of fat. However, if you're active, having one tablespoon of olive oil a day is okay. That's actually quite a generous amount that goes a long way. Nut butters, including coconut butter, provide the creamy mouth feel but have more body, as well as more nutrients, since they contain the nut's original fiber—which also makes their fat less concentrated.

Limit dairy

Dairy is a category of foods most people can benefit from eliminating from their normal diet. This doesn't mean it has to be excluded completely and avoided like the plague, unless you have a specific allergy.

I personally keep dairy in the "occasional exceptions/treats" category. This means I don't use dairy products or buy them, but occasionally I will indulge.

Occasional dairy treats for me would be something like Italian eggplant parmeggiano, or gelato — each contains only just enough cheese or milk for flavor.

If I'm traveling to Greece, I'm not going to say no to real Greek yogurt with fruit — a true treat.

I think considering dairy an occasional treat or indulgence is healthy. I've noticed that the dairy products that affect me the most negatively are loads of cheese on something like pizza. So here's one place I would make an exception to my general rule of "eating whatever is offered when invited" and "eating whatever I feel like on vacation."

So far my hosts haven't offered to make pizza, so I haven't had this issue, but this is where I would probably suggest the possibility of eating something else.

But other foods that contain a small quantity of dairy eaten only on occasion have not affected my health negatively. Listen to your own body's responses and decide where your tolerance lies.

Limit wheat

As a whole grain, wheat has some good qualities. The ancient Greeks made extra efforts to produce wheat, even though barley was easier to grow in their soil. Ever since, wheat has been venerated as a staple food in Western societies and beyond. Obviously, it provides a good source of carbohydrate calories, as well as fiber. It also contains a good amount of protein, B vitamins, and some minerals, such as magnesium and manganese.

However, for the most part you're not going to be eating wheat as a virtuous whole grain. In its more common guise as a refined flour (sometimes retrofitted with the nutrients stripped from it in the refinement process), it is almost ubiquitous in prepared food.

Now, common sense says it would never have gotten this ubiquitous if it hadn't worked for great numbers of people over thousands of years. On the other hand, this long use has led to some changes to the wheat itself. Wheat contains more gluten than any other grain, which means it's easier to make the dough hold together for bread, convenient and portable. This is why it's been prized for so long.

And since ancient times, people have been cross-breeding wheat to have even more gluten. The older strains of wheat still exist. You can get them at the health food store: kamut, spelt, einkorn, emmer, triticale... Many people with wheat sensitivities tolerate these grains better.

And that's because modern wheat contains *even more* gluten, as well as another starch, called amylopectin A, which makes baked goods fluffy and has a striking effect on blood sugar levels *even in wholegrain bread*. Wheat also contains more gliadin than it used to, another protein like gluten to which many people are sensitive. Gluten itself can be very inflammatory in the gut. The most severe version of this is celiac disease, whose sufferers must avoid all gluten-containing grains but will suffer most severely if they accidentally consume some wheat. However, many people who do not have celiac still suffer from inflammation if they consume wheat.

Proteins in wheat also break down in the gut and bind to the opioid receptors in the brain—in other words, the body recognizes them as opium-like substances! No wonder some people are so addicted to wheat.

Bear this information in mind as you make your own decisions around wheat. You may already know that you need to avoid it completely, whether because it makes you sick or because you tend to get addicted to it. Otherwise, find your comfort level. Perhaps you'll eat it occasionally at social gatherings but keep it out of your home. Perhaps you'll make your own bread using the heritage wheats mentioned above. Whatever you do, the advice to limit consumption of *modern* wheat is very sound.

If you eat animal protein, focus on fish and lean meat

Many ex-raw foodists get convinced they need animal protein in their diet, but they don't want to start eating flesh. So they go heavy in the dairy and egg department. Eating dairy as a source of nutrients can be extremely problematic, and "raw" dairy is no exception. See dairy as something you could eat occasionally as a treat rather than a food that you have on an ongoing basis.

The jury is still out on eggs. I know there are many degrees of opinion on eggs, but I personally will stick with the scientific consensus on the topic.

We know that high quantities of saturated fats and cholesterol in the diet can raise blood cholesterol levels and that this can be a factor contributing to heart disease. Eggs are particularly rich in in cholesterol.

On the other hand, lean meat and fish can be quite reasonable in saturated fat and cholesterol levels. Many plant foods actually contain as much or more saturated fat than some animal foods.

Food	Cholesterol	Saturated Fat
2 eggs	420 mg.	4 g.
1 filet salmon (6 ounces)	108 mg.	4 g.
1 filet cod (4 ounces)	43 mg.	0 g. (trace amounts probably exist)
6 ounces grass-fed beef (lean) (210 g.)	118 mg.	2 g.
Coconut milk (1/2 cup)	0 mg.	25 g.
Almonds, 2 ounces	0 mg.	2 g.
Avocado, 1 Hass	0 mg.	4 g.

Because the current scientific consensus is to limit cholesterol intake and limit saturated fat intake to less than 5% of calories, and also because no long-lived culture was really much dairy- and egg-eating, it makes more sense if you're going to eat animal protein to focus mainly on clean fish and some meat, with dairy or eggs being used occasionally as a treat.

If You Eat Fish, Eat Clean Fish

Some would claim that no fish is unpolluted, and they are all contaminated to some degree. But the real questions are "How much is too much?" and "Where are you getting the fish from?"

If you decide to eat fish, it's important to know where you're getting your fish from and not simply to purchase what's available. There's a dramatic difference in the quality of wild salmon as opposed to farm-raised "Atlantic" salmon, which is damaged by extensive use of antibiotics and can be high in PCBs, a significant endocrine disruptor that may be carcinogenic.

Some cities like Vancouver have a program (called SeaChoice in Vancouver) where restaurants can agree to serve and identify on their menu sustainable fish choices — those that don't encourage overfishing and bad farming practice. Check in your area if there's a similar program.

High quality fish is available; you just have to look harder for it. In some cases, you may have to mail-order it (frozen, of course!).

Limit red meat

Opinions on animal protein vary greatly, and the emotional thermometer around this issue runs high. There are plenty of arguments are on both sides.

I have looked at the evidence presented both by people who recommend a 100% vegan diet, and those who advocate some animal foods.

The only absolute that seems to be proven at this point is that a plant-based diet is a requirement for optimal health. The words "plant-based" in this context mean: where most of your calories come from plants.

The only people that disagree with this view are proponents of the Atkins diet, and of Aajonus Vonderplanitz' Primal diet, and some other paleo and primal diets, who recommend getting a majority of calories from animal foods, as was supposedly the case in the ancient history of humankind.

The fiercest critics of animal food consumption, such as T. Colin Campbell, agree that 10% of calories is the upper limit above which animal food consumption may pose a considerable health risk. Dr. Joel Fuhrman also comes to the same conclusion.

If we look at many healthy cultures around the world, meat is viewed as a condiment or an occasional treat, not a daily staple.

The real question of interest for us is really whether a small but regular intake of animal products can bring benefits.

Some vegans reading this book will remain vegans. The ethical considerations are just too strong for them to even consider eating some animal products.

When it comes to red meat, eating it a maximum of once or twice a week is probably the right frequency. If other sources of animal protein are consumed, like fish, then you will stay around or under the 10% limit established by even the most convinced anti-animal protein researchers.

Matching Food to Activity Level

With the hype that surrounds diets and weight loss programs, some important considerations get lost along the way. For example, let's take the "war on sugar" in all its forms.

It's fashionable now to hate sugar with a passion and blame it for the epidemic of obesity, among other things. Some authors even argue that the sugar in fruit is "almost as bad" as the refined sugar in other foods.

All of these authors explain how sugar has taken over our diets in recent years; especially high fructose corn syrup, which is now used to sweeten a number of things, like beverages, tomato ketchup, and pretty much any variety of prepared foods. But along with this refined sugar, consumption of refined carbs such as white bread and products made with flour, has jumped in recent decades. Some authors even lump the humble potato, because it is white, along with other "evil" carbs like white bread and white sugar. Poor potato — full of fiber, potassium and other nutrients, is being lumped with the bad guys, just because of its color. Call it food racism?

The reality is that refined sugar in itself is not a poison or a bad thing. The glucose and fructose extracted from the sugar cane or corn kernels is the same glucose or fructose that is found in fruit and other foods, and refined sugar contains similar sugars to those the body ends up with after digesting starches. The sugar is the same, but there's a whole lot of stuff missing: fiber, vitamins, water, minerals, etc.

Because of this, some authors actually claim that "all sugar is the same." Once digested, the sugar that comes from digesting the starch in the potato is just as bad as the white sugar people put in their coffee. This concept is, of course, ludicrous. Starch digests slowly, and vegetables or whole grains containing it are full of fiber, which slows down absorption further, and provides other benefits.

Even refined sugar is not evil in every single context. The problem is that we have a population that is extremely inactive, but eats massive amounts of food, as if in training for a marathon!

Speaking of marathons, long-distance runners know that simple sugars are essential to their success. Before a race, and during training periods lasting more than 90 minutes, products containing refined sugars are frequently consumed, and they are perfectly utilized by the body. After a workout, glycogen (stored carbohydrate) reserves are depleted, and must be replenished quickly. Therefore, in this context, eating foods that have a high glycemic index actually makes sense. There are times when raising your blood sugar *quickly* is desirable.

Food intake has to match activity levels. And in modern times, in Western societies, the problem is that food intake doesn't match activity levels, which is why people slowly but surely gain weight every year, or develop metabolic disorders such as type-2 diabetes.

Modern diet gurus have gone to an extreme and demonized one category of food, because it's much easier to teach that than try to teach a more balanced way of living. And they are always right in a certain *context*, but not in all contexts.

Diet	Food Demons
Raw vegan diet	Cooked foods. Fats.
Low-Fat Plant-Based Diet	Animal foods. Fats.
Modern Paleo Diet	Carbohydrates. Sugar.
Four Hour Body Diet	Grains, fruit.

Take sugar, for example. There are times when I consume refined sugar. One example could be as an occasional treat. I have a friend who really enjoys drinking Italian sodas (San Pellegrino). So on rare occasions, I'll have one. Those occasions will be accompanied by long days of hiking or on days I'll be running. The extra sugar coursing through my bloodstream will not just be sitting there; I'll be using it. So in this context, refined sugar is not that bad. Of course, I wouldn't want to be using it as my main source of energy. I'm talking about an occasional exception.

Another example: if I was going to be running a half marathon on a hot sunny day, I wouldn't hesitate to drink some Gatorade or other commercial "sports drink" at some point during the race. In this context, the salt contained in the sports drink will be utilized by my body, and will actually be useful. The refined carbs in the drink will be burned off.

Granted, Gatorade is not a health drink. In fact, you could make the effort to produce a healthier alternative, juicing celery and whatnot, and mixing it with date water. But in the context of a race, the quality of the ingredients actually doesn't matter that much, because your body is really only using the raw materials. It may actually be much more convenient to drink the Gatorade provided at the event than to bring your own drink, adding to your weight and maybe even slowing you down during the race when you pull it out. So let's say I'm running a half marathon a few times a year, and drink some commercial sports drinks during these events, is my health going to be negatively affected? Absolutely not. Not in this context, where the substance consumed matches the activity level. I'm making rational decisions based on consideration of all factors.

In other contexts, drinking Gatorade doesn't make sense. It's a "sports drink," yet people drink it as a refreshing beverage when they're inactive. Can you see how context makes all the difference?

Let's take oil, another refined food. For many years, I spoke out against the use of oils (for example, olive oil), following the lead of many vegan experts such as Dr. John McDougall and others. I had one caveat though: I explained in my books that one could use a small amount of olive oil on occasion, if they liked the taste in salads, as long as they didn't overdo it in the fat department elsewhere.

Oil is an interesting food, because it's marketed as a health food, yet is just as refined as refined sugar. Once an olive is pressed, the fiber and most of the nutrients are gone (except a few vitamins). But fat is a more complex nutrient than sugar. Different types of fat act differently in the body. Saturated fats are considered "bad" because they raise cholesterol levels. Monounsaturated fats, like what's mostly contained in olive oils, do not have that effect. And certain types of polyunsaturated fats, such as the famous omega 3 fats, actually lower the bad LDL cholesterol and raise the good HDL cholesterol, while providing other benefits too.

But what all oils have in common is that they are concentrated sources of calories. One tablespoon of oil contains more calories (120 to be exact) than any other food. Refined sugar is only 50 calories per tablespoon.

When oil is used copiously in preparation of food, the overall caloric value of the food is much higher, and since it's not buffered by any additional fiber, the food is richer. But at the same time, the dressing causes the greens to wilt down, so it's easier to eat more. Most people don't eat less of it because it's richer. Even if they did, it would have to be a lot less in order to offset the increase in calories, or a lot of the oil would have to remain unconsumed at the bottom of the bowl!

In other words, if you add a couple of tablespoons of oil to your salad, you're likely to eat as much salad as if you had a fat-free dressing. But the salad with oil will contain 240 calories more.

Since one of the good things about greens is that they contain fat-soluble vitamins like vitamin K, it is actually a good idea to eat some fat with your salad, and even low-fat diet proponents are recommending this. But it can be accomplished with a few slices of avocado, or a small drizzle of olive oil.

Too much fat in the bloodstream also impairs insulin function and lowers insulin sensitivity, rendering you more sensitive to carbohydrate, which can have the effect of raising insulin and blood sugar levels. Over time on a diet both high in fat and high in sugar or refined carbs, and combined with an inactive lifestyle, this can lead to diabetes.

But let's put it in perspective. If you're active and at your ideal weight, using one or two tablespoons of olive oil per day (on a 2500 or 3000 calorie diet), in the context of a whole foods, plant-based diet, is not going to be a problem. One tablespoon is actually quite a generous amount, and can give a lot of taste to stir-fries and other dishes.

For years, I cooked everything without oil. But more recently, I noticed how unsatisfied I was with some of my meals. I work out five or six times a week and I try to stay active by walking a lot as well. My caloric needs are close to 3500 calories a day, almost twice as many calories as some of my female readers might need.

So in my case, a little olive oil is really not a problem — especially considering the fact that I don't eat more than an ounce of nuts a day, and don't eat many fatty foods in general.

So when I make a stir-fry, I may use 1 tablespoon of oil. The amount of food I make will be enough for two meals, so the amount of oil consumed will be 60 calories-worth per meal. That's nothing, in my context.

In the context of a weight loss program, oil can be a problem. It can quickly add unnecessary calories.

So as you can see, context makes a big difference with some dietary choices. It's not that certain foods are inherently evil, but they are just used improperly and in the wrong context, and usually in the wrong quantities, too.

Social issues

By far, the biggest complaint that I've heard from people who have attempted to live on a raw food diet have to do with difficulties incorporating this lifestyle into the social world at large. The only way to really make it work is to create an alternate reality, where many of the normal interactions of life are either avoided or masterfully handled to avoid bringing up issues around your refusing to eat "normal" food and drinks. Many manage to do it well for a few years, but most eventually find it difficult to maintain a 100% raw food diet without alienating too many friends and family members.

It's possible to do, but usually it requires a complete rethinking of your life and your priorities, along with great self-confidence and social skills. But one thing that's unavoidable, and probably one of the biggest social drawbacks of a raw food diet is that it shrinks the menu of options in life when it comes to certain choices, such as where to travel, whom to spend time with, and sometimes even whom to choose as a life partner.

I didn't personally realize the extent to which my raw food or vegan diet had alienated me from the rest of the world and "social possibilities" until I made a conscious decision that I would no longer insist on eating my perfect diet in all circumstances. Once I started living with this more flexible diet, I realized how my social interactions had totally changed. I reconnected with friends I hadn't spent much quality time with, and I also made dramatic progress in many aspects of my life through those new connections and rekindled friendships.

For example, during the winter of 2012-2013 I went for a week-long vacation to an island in the Caribbean with a friend. On the island where we were, there was no possibility of eating a raw food diet and very little possibility of eating a vegan diet. But I had already made the decision that this trip was very important to me and that diet was secondary; finding the perfect foods would not be my focus. In the end, it turned out to be one of the best and most positive weeks of my life.

It can be tricky to manage the balance between "cheating" and keeping strong and solid health principles, but it's doable. The reward can be a more successful and balanced life that is not just focused on managing a diet.

Many of my readers, in anticipation of this book, wrote me about this particular topic:

> So happy that you are doing books that incorporate both raw and cooked foods. I cannot begin to tell you how much closer I am with my family now that I join them for meals (I have the vegan courses) and have not isolated myself with an all raw diet. I am seen so many health benefits since I began my 80% raw, 20% cooked food diet. And now, I can influence my family to eat healthier. When I ate 100% raw, they felt I was judging them for their choices, which put so much distance between us. I'd rather eat raw and cooked and have the love of my family. Thank you Fred for all your guidance and support. Gavin R

> --

> As a businessman on frequent conference and business trips, I found it difficult to actually eat 100% raw, although I did so for two years. It wore me out. The effort and stress of swimming against the stream became a grind that outweighed the benefits.

> --

> My experience as a raw foodist was mixed: at first I had loads of energy, clear skin, cellulite disappeared, no body odor. On the other hand, I experienced social isolation due to my raw diet. One friend got really upset with me because I declined the cake he cooked. Also, I worked in the office and really felt the lack of oxygen and sunshine like never before. I was hungry all the time towards the end of my raw year and became extremely thin. I also experienced excruciating pain in my spine and joints and dehydrated skin. I ate mostly fresh fruit with minimum fat like in 80-10-10 program, no greens or dried fruit. Eventually I had to give up being 100% raw and even though I still eat a lot of raw food, I'm no longer dogmatic about it.

Ultimately, it's a matter of priorities and values. It can be that maintaining a raw food diet or a vegan diet is your number one priority in life. There's nothing wrong with that in itself.

However, pay attention to the difference between dogmatically holding on to a principle that doesn't fully serve you and truly doing the right thing for you. If eating a 100% raw vegan diet all the time is the *right* thing for you at most levels of your life, you should make the necessary compromises to maintain it. If you find that it's probably an ideal that doesn't fully serve you, then create new rules that will liberate you. As one of my readers wrote me, the "effort and stress of swimming against the stream" can become a grind that outweighs the benefits."

Restaurants

Restaurants can be tricky on a raw food diet, or any diet, for that matter. When I was eating 100% raw, I avoided restaurants almost entirely. I occasionally ate at raw food restaurants, but because the food served there is usually based on nuts and seeds and very high in fat, I wouldn't feel very good afterwards.

Even when I was eating close to 100% raw but with occasional exceptions, I avoided restaurants. When my dad was alive, he loved to eat out for brunch with my brother and me every other Sunday. I would usually order a fruit plate or smoothie, which was rather unsatisfying because the fruit was rarely as ripe or good as I would have liked — but it didn't matter because I was there to spend time with my family. I would occasionally order some oatmeal, or buckwheat pancakes (made with 100% buckwheat flour — a French Canadian dish).

People have made various suggestions for raw foodists who want to know what to do when they find themselves in a situation where they have to eat at a restaurant for business, or in other social settings. Some people suggested simply pretending you have already eaten, but having a glass of something like orange juice with your group. Others have suggested calling the restaurant in advance to request a special meal, or even pretending to the waiter that you have food allergies. I also knew a raw foodist who carried a little card with her listing all the items she was allowed to eat, and asked the waiter to pass it along to the chef and ask if they could do something with it. One raw foodist I know ordered a salad once — but found it too small, so requested another one "three times the size." Many raw foodists simply eat beforehand, and then order something small, like a green salad with dressing on the side (which they won't touch) to avoid being difficult or looking too weird. In some cases, they bring their own dressings.

These are all hidden admissions that it's very difficult to follow a raw food diet in social situations, unless you lie, or go out of your way to make a special request that probably won't be accommodated the way you would like.

All of these inconveniences are generally not a big issue for most people, but can contribute to the feeling of social alienation many people feel when eating a 100% raw food diet. It's not that most people miss eating out at restaurants, but they also cannot eat out with friends in other circumstances, share a drink, and otherwise feel part of the "normal world."

Some people don't mind any of this because of their personality and feeling that they are doing the right thing for their health — which is their priority. I certainly think that this attitude is great, as long as you are happy with the choices you make and options available to you.

In my case, I rarely find myself at a restaurant, so I've decided I will not make a big fuss about what I eat on those rare occasions. I'm usually the one to invite people over for dinner, and people are happy to eat and enjoy the healthy meals I prepare. The few times I eat out are occasionally at home with friends or business associates. The other times would be when I'm traveling abroad, and having some meals at restaurants is the only convenient option.

In the past, I had clear rules for eating out — and I'm not even talking about raw foods. Eating 100% raw vegan at a restaurant is extremely difficult — especially if you intend this meal to actually nourish you and not leave you hungry half an hour later. Having a vegan meal is possible in most places, but what I have found is that it's next to impossible to make sure the meal meets my *ideal* standards, such as being low in oil and salt, and having enough vegetables. I would often explain exactly what I wanted, only to be disappointed when I received my plate.

What I have discovered is that often the vegan option at a restaurant is *not* the healthiest choice. Often the vegan option is a pasta dish, or another dish containing a lot of refined carbs. I now find it better to simply look for the *healthiest* dish on the menu, and order that — whether it's vegan or not. In some cases, that would be a vegetarian dish including some small amount of dairy (e.g. cheese on top, which could even be picked off if you wanted). In other cases, it might be fish. I know this philosophy will not work for some of my readers because they feel very strongly about vegan ethics — but it works for me.

An example comes from a recent trip around the world I took with my then-wife. When we were in the Philippines, we found it very difficult to find healthy foods at restaurants. And whenever we made special requests, people didn't really understand what we wanted. It turned out that whatever vegan choices (or special requests) we could make at restaurants were much more unhealthy than the standard choices. Pasta would come out overcooked, doused in a very sweet sauce; and vegetables were fried. In this situation, it would have been better to simply order a straightforward, non-vegan meal, such as grilled fish and rice.

I also drink socially, and I find this is a great way to feel part of social situations without having to make other unhealthy choices. For example if everyone is drinking wine at a family gathering, then I will have a glass of wine. Enjoying an occasional drink with friends is a great social bond — especially when you feel that other aspects of your diet or lifestyle may restrict your social choices. In some cases, it's perfectly fine to meet someone at a restaurant and only order a glass of wine, and maybe something simple like a salad. This is always a no-fuss option that makes it really easy to blend in any social situations at restaurants, business meetings and family gatherings.

In North American cultures, people are quite used to special dietary requests. Many people don't drink, only drink decaf coffee, avoid gluten, are vegetarian, or have other special dietary needs. Therefore it is not completely out of place to refuse something that's offered to you in social situations when you have dietary or other restrictions.

In other cultures — especially Asian ones — it's considered very rude to refuse to taste food or drink offered by your guests. Many North Americans don't understand that concept, but it's quite prevalent in many parts of the world. I knew a raw foodist who was a businessman in Asia. He ate a raw food diet most of the time, but had to make an exception when he was doing business in China — because he simply could not refuse to taste food and drinks offered by his hosts. If he had done so, it would have been considered extremely rude by his business associates — and he would have lost the business.

In North America and to some degree Europe, and other Western countries like Australia, dietary restrictions are common, but rarely are people confronted with someone who literally cannot have *anything* on the menu. Some raw foodists take their diet to such an extreme that they will refuse to even have a cup of herbal tea, or eat a salad that has a little olive oil on it. I have found that most people in restaurants and other hosts in social situations are quite happy to accommodate, but because they have never encountered such a level of dietary restriction before, they are very likely not to get it right, even if you explain clearly. Someone might ask for a salad with no dressing, but find that the salad has a bit of olive oil on it. You might return it, but in some situations — such as business dealings — you can be viewed in a negative light by your colleagues, who won't be able to relate to your obsession over small details.

What to Order at a Restaurant

Some restaurant options are better than others, and choosing these can help remove some of the stress of eating out, allowing you to enjoy the occasion without feeling sick or guilty afterwards. While restaurant food is rarely "healthy," it's possible to stick to a few safe choices. I will list the most commonly found and the healthiest — whether they are vegan or not.

It may help you to have a few simple rules about what "not to eat" at a restaurant or other social occasions. Everyone will be different in this regard, so I won't give you rules that you should imperatively follow. It's more about how you react to certain foods (gluten, dairy, etc.) and your personal values (vegan, etc.).

Here are my rules that I try to follow when eating out:

- Avoid big doses of dairy (cheese, creamy sauces, etc.).
- Avoid fried foods, as well as anything that includes the word "crispy" or "creamy."
- Avoid oily foods.
- Avoid appetizers. Only order main courses or salad.
- Avoid soups (too salty and not satisfying).
- Avoid dessert (this rule is occasionally broken for a "once in a life-time" dessert experience).
- Avoid anything in a sauce or dressing, and if necessary request it "on the side"

Other rules that others might find useful include:

- Avoid big doses of gluten (like bread, pasta), but stay flexible with gluten-containing condiments like soy sauce.
- Avoid meat, animal products.

In general, American sit-down chain restaurants (TGI Friday's, Olive Garden, Applebee's, etc.) tend to have the worst and unhealthiest food, disguised in an appearance of wholesomeness. Next are regular fast food chains (McDonald's, Wendy's, Subway, etc.) although they are much less unhealthy than the bigger chain restaurants. Your best bets are family-owned or non-franchised ethnic restaurants, especially:

Mexican

It's best to order soft tortillas, which are baked instead of fried. Corn tortillas are a healthier choice as well. Salsa is tasty, and look for black beans. You can order grilled fish and marinated veggies.

Thai

Here are some creative Thai ideas. Order Summer Rolls. They are not fried, and are filled with veggies and rice noodles. Order Tom Yum soup made with mushrooms, broth, and lemongrass. You can often get this with tofu or with lean meat or fish. Thai restaurants usually have a grilled fish choice. Curries are a good choice as well, although high in (coconut) fat.

Japanese

Japanese restaurants have a wide array of dishes for vegetarians. From sushi to cooked vegetable stir fries, it's rare to find a Japanese restaurant that doesn't satisfy the vegetarian or health-conscious palate.

Vietnamese

Dishes in Vietnamese restaurants may be steamed, fried, or simmered, and usually include rice or noodles. A number of dishes are naturally low in fat, but be sure to ask about preparation methods if you are in doubt. Here are some tips for making healthy choices at Vietnamese restaurants.

Good Choices:
- steamed or simmered dishes
- Vegetarian Pho soup
- salads rolls or summer rolls
- Vietnamese bouillabaisse
- grilled vegetable skewers

Grilled vegetables on skewers are a good alternative to traditional barbecued spareribs. Caramel sauce is typically listed as nuoc duong thang on Vietnamese menus. Be on the lookout for it. It is high in sugar. Dishes that have been simmered may sound healthy, but the addition of this sugary sauce makes them less so. Look for soups that contain lots of vegetables, and leave off the deep-fried choices. The Pho soups (made with broth from fish, meat, or vegetables) typically come with a side of fresh greens, herbs, and bean sprouts, which you can add to the broth as you eat it so that they gently steam.

Greek

Many people think of Greek food as healthy, but you still have to pay attention to what you order. Many Greek restaurants saturate foods in butter and cook with high-fat red meats. Here are a few of the healthier choices you'll see on the menu.

Souvlaki are grilled kebabs made of chicken, lamb, or pork. Avoid large servings of rice or pita bread and ask for steamed veggies or a side salad instead.

Horiatiki Salata is the name for Greek garden salad. When you order a Greek salad, you can ask for no feta, and dressing on the side. For extra flavor, ask for a side of tzatziki sauce. Tzatziki is Greek yogurt flavored with mint, cucumber and garlic. It's not enough dairy to worry about.

Who doesn't love hummus? Hummus is a chickpea-based dip made with tahini (sesame seed paste), garlic, lemon juice, olive oil, and other spices. Many restaurants offer hummus in a variety of flavors including roasted red pepper, spinach and artichoke, and roasted garlic. Chickpeas are rich in protein and have a glycemic index of 12, meaning hummus will satiate your appetite without loading you down with extra calories. When ordering, ask for plenty of fresh vegetables for dipping. Typically hummus is served with warm pita bread, cucumbers and tomatoes.

Kakavia soup is a traditional Greek fisherman's soup typically made with the catch of the day, or whatever is seasonal, like snapper, mullet, or whitefish. Chefs may also add in shellfish like lobster and shrimp for added flavor. Loaded with heart-healthy vegetables and herbs, a bowl of this soup provides an excellent source of vitamins and antioxidants.

Melitzanosalata is a dip of ground eggplant, tahini, garlic, and olive oil. It's a great source of heart-healthy ingredients. Ask for extra veggies on the side for dipping so you don't fill up on pita bread.

Since Greek food is steeped in the Mediterranean tradition, many Greek restaurant menus offer a variety of seafood meals. Look for a dish that is grilled, pan-seared, or broiled; not fried, and offers a side of fresh vegetables or salad.

Indian

Indian restaurant menus can be a challenge, especially if you don't understand the language. However, Indian menu items can be healthy. Many of the items are made with rice, grains, and vegetables. Some are also made with a lot of oil. You can easily choose healthier options if you have a clear understanding of what to look for and what to avoid. Here are some tips.

Since many of the appetizers are fried, you can skip them and move onto the main course.

Try Gobhi Matar Tamatar, a vegetarian dish that will provide you with plenty of healthy vegetables. The dish is composed of cauliflower, peas and tomatoes.

Avoid fried or fat-soaked breads. Many of the bread options at Indian restaurants have been fried or soaked in fat, such as kulcha, poori and and roti. You can choose healthier breads, like naan, which is typically baked, or chapatti, which is cooked on a dry griddle.

The papadam that usually comes out with the appetizers is bread made from fiber-rich lentils. It can be baked, but at restaurants it is generally fried.

Choose items on the menu containing the word tandoori. Items flagged tandoori have been cooked in a tandoori oven. The tandoori oven cooks foods at high temperatures in a way similar to a traditional Italian pizza oven.

Choose items from the vegetarian menu. Choose vegetarian entrees made with lentils and beans ("dal" denotes a lentil stew). Also, find menu items made with green vegetables, such as spinach. Items with green vegetables usually contain the word saag or palak.

Traditional Italian

Let's be honest. When we think of health-conscious cuisine for vegetarians, not too many of us would put Italian food at the top of the list. Many people think there are no healthy foods in Italian restaurants. But there are, so keep reading!

Minestrone soup is a good way to start out a meal in an Italian restaurant. And follow it with a salad. Order the dressing on the side. For your main course, if you eat animal protein, you can order fish or chicken. I think with Italian food it's really a matter of HOW the food is prepared, and Italian restaurants in general are very amenable to preparing your food any way you like it. It's easy for them!

I know you are going to order the pasta. You've been lusting after it ever since your friend announced a gathering at the Italian restaurant, right? After all, what's the point of going to an Italian restaurant if not to eat pasta? There are so many varieties of pasta, pasta sauces, and fillings for ravioli that I'm sure you can find something you'll enjoy.

Just remember the basics: avoid creamy sauces, Alfredo, large amounts of cheese, too much bread, and heavy dressings. When in doubt, ask what the dish contains. You can enjoy your experience when you take a few minutes to figure out what's best to order.

Most other restaurants that are popular are either French or have a French-inspired menu. Any chef working in a non-ethnic restaurant in America or most of Europe (and, in fact, the rest of the developed world) will have been trained at a cooking school, and most cooking schools are based on French cuisine, which has been the most influential in the world. French cuisine can be delicious and very refined, but it is generally not healthy, with all the heavy sauces, extreme amounts of butter, and small portions of concentrated, fatty food. That's why ethnic restaurants are generally safer and healthier options.

The Importance of Being Part of the Social World

You can decide to be part of the world, or you can decide to live in a world of your own. Either way is fine — as long as it's your choice and you're happy with it, rather than feeling forced into it by the implications of your diet.

What I've discovered over the years is, humans are humans. Whether you eat a raw food diet or you eat fried chicken with fries, you're still a human being, probably with the same flaws, emotional challenges, and demons. I've noticed that within the raw food movement, the same drama, competition, back-stabbing, gossip, envy, hatred, and love stories abound as in the world at large. You would think that raw foodists would somehow be exempt from this or have transcended this, but it seems to be part of the human condition, no matter what we choose to eat. Diet is just one part of life, and it doesn't seem to affect the other parts as much as you would think.

Also, raw foodists can't reject society at large. At some point, you have to interact with people who have a vastly different lifestyle from you. If you have children, you already know how true this is.

It's not "us vs. them." There's a way to blend in without having to follow the path everyone else is following. You can be a unique individual and decide to live your life the way you want, but also interact with the rest of the world and move freely between different groups of people, like water over rocks.

Real World Issues: Dieting With a Partner

One reader recently sent me this email:

> I used to be 100% raw but now I'm 80% raw because I find that I can eat healthier without the pressure of being raw all the time. I prefer raw foods, but my partner prefers to eat healthy cooked vegan foods,
>
> The largest impediments I find to going completely raw are social and being involved in a relationship with someone who is not. I have been steadily increasing the amount of raw food as a percentage of my whole diet over the past few years. My body is gradually wanting and needing more raw food. This approach is better for me than committing to 100% because then I fall off the wagon and binge.
>
> The biggest problem for me is living with others who eat a cooked food diet, the smell is alluring. Also I find raw food difficult socially.

Finding a partner who eats the same diet as you do can be difficult, especially if you choose to follow a 100% raw or vegan diet (or both). Add children to the mix, and it can prove even more challenging.

My experience dating raw vegan women

I didn't think I was going to share about my love life in this book, but this little bit of insight from my 15 years of experience in the raw food world might be useful to some.

Over the years, I've noticed that a disproportionate number of women are interested in the raw food diet. About 82% of my readers are women. This means that overall, fewer men are interested in veganism, raw foodism or a healthy lifestyle than women. As a man, this can be great news if you're interested in dating a raw vegan woman, because the odds will be in your favor, so to speak. But for women, this is not such great news because odds are that they will not find a man who shares the same beliefs about diet, or has the same interest in following along.

By the way, I know that political correctness would require me to translate all my heterosexual talk here into every possible combination of male and female relationships, but I think the situation is clear enough for everybody to get my point.

So where does *my* love life fit into this? Like I said, significantly more women are interested in the raw food diet than men. So that's why for many years I had no trouble dating women who shared my lifestyle, and this led to a few long-term relationships, including a marriage that ended in 2012.

What I discovered is that the issue is not so much with diet as with compatibility. That's why I decided I no longer want to date raw vegan women exclusively. First of all, I'm not really a pure raw vegan. I'm not a strict vegan, and I don't eat a 100% raw food diet. So raw vegan women who insist on a partner who eats like them wouldn't find the right match in me.

Obviously, I prefer to be with someone who shares similar values when it comes to diet; however it's no longer one of my top priorities as far as relationships are concerned. Certainly, I want to be with a healthy, health-conscious person; but perfect compatibility in diet is not a huge requirement for me anymore.

Someone looking for a partner who insists on very clear dietary criteria (like vegan, or raw foods) will ultimately reduce their options. This can be good because sometimes a smaller niche means that two people may find each other more easily, but it can also lead to disappointment. Most people don't follow exactly the same diet throughout their life, and as one partner changes, the strong bond the two had in common may get broken.

I don't want you to read between the lines and assume this is necessary what happened to me. But in my experience it is a very common mistake to choose a person because of some common values while overlooking bigger aspects of personality and compatibility, which have nothing to do with diet.

Men will generally have few problems finding a woman interested in eating better and open to dietary changes. Women will find it more difficult to find a man who shares the same interests, or to convince a man to change his diet without causing some resentment.

The best approach I've found for women is to not try to change her man. Instead, she tries to be an indirect influence by sharing how dietary changes made her feel, rather than trying to change the other person. I've seen many successful relationships where women had partners who did not eat like them, but eventually agreed to make some changes. The most important thing is that you are with the right person, and diet is a detail that can often easily be handled.

Many couples decide on a "core" menu that appeals to both, such as raw foods, salads, fruit, whole grains, etc., and then create some add-ons for the person that may eat differently (e.g. pasta, or grilled meat). Agreeing on a core menu that is healthy and tasty, and then adding the missing items that the other person can't live without, is an easy compromise to make. But compromises go both ways, and you may also have to loosen some of your principles, as we've discussed at length in this book, to make it work.

Existing relationships, where an established pattern of eating together has already been solidified, and is being shaken by one person's desire to change their diet, are more difficult. The best approach is a gradual one. Because you are the person changing, it would be unfair to expect the structure of your entire family's meals to change overnight. Gradually, it will be possible to create a workable menu for both people.

A word of advice for women: don't underestimate the impact of male psychology in this area. Universally, men hate to have their partners impose changes. It's not that men are necessarily reluctant to change, but rather that they abhor "guilt trips" and being told what to do. Make these dietary changes seductive rather than implying deprivation. The old saying "the way to a man's heart is through his stomach" should be the guiding principle; so make sure you find a few good recipes for him to try, even if they are not exactly what you would personally eat. A delicious raw food dessert, even if it's not healthy, will do a lot more to open a man's mind to the *possibility* of trying out a higher-raw diet than a bowl of fruit or a smoothie. Once he's hooked on the first bite, it will be easier to feed him what you really want him to eat.

Psychology and a little seduction are important when encouraging your partner to make some changes in their life. Remember, you are the one who changed first — you're the disturbing agent. Most people don't like to be moved from their comfort zone. So don't push them out of it; rather, entice them to take a step out on their own.

Families with Children

When raising children, it's a challenge to know what to teach them about food.

So while as adults we may have a way of eating that follows certain "rules," I feel it's important to expose children to as many food choices as possible and see how their palates develop. They are not miniature versions of us; they will have their own preferences. Have them try all kinds of fruits and vegetables. Try all different ethnic foods. Teach them how to feel comfortable in the kitchen. Make food fun and make it an adventure. Eating and enjoying food can involve plenty of teaching moments, but don't make it all so serious. There's a time and a place for food politics. And help them learn that not all people make the same choices around food and nutrition. This will help them not be so judgmental about what's "right and wrong" about food. It will help them relax and develop their own palates.

Think about it! We all have some food we didn't like that our parents pushed on us. I'll bet you still can't eat that food to this day. And maybe there are some days your kid wants to sit down to a whole cucumber? Let them go for it; enjoy your kids and their journey with food. I'm sure you'll even find some foods they'll help YOU enjoy!

Common Problems and Their Causes

By reviewing the stories of ex-raw foodists (and sometimes ex-vegans), I have identified a few common problems people run into.

Sometimes, they were able to solve these problems with proper supplementation, or a different raw vegan diet (such as a low-fat one), but the problems below affected people who did not find any improvement from supplementation or (for some who tried it) low-fat veganism.

Of course, this is purely anecdotal and it's impossible to decide exactly what *actually* happened (versus what they said happened) in every case. However, I believe it would be a little close-minded to totally dismiss these stories as happening in "anorexic" people who "didn't do the diet properly."

Dental Problems

This mostly affects raw-foodists, who tend to have more dental problems than the general population. I discussed the reasons in my book *Raw Food Controversies*.

Essentially, the low caloric density of the diet encourages frequent snacking on sugary foods (like fruit), which promotes decay. Eliminating snacking and eating actual meals is a key element in preventing dental problems on a raw food diet. Strict dental hygiene is required as well.

Some vegans report an increase in dental decay on a vegan diet, but I suspect that's simply because they're eating more refined carbohydrates like flour, cookies, and vegan junk foods. For more information on the topic, please consult my book *Raw Food Controversies*.

Low Sex Drive

This symptom is very common, but tends to only appear in men following low-fat raw diets of fruits and vegetables, with minimal or no nuts and seeds. Many of these raw foodists, mainly young men, experience a complete disappearance of their normal sex drive after a short period on the diet. Most of these men, and some women, find themselves losing interest in sex. A raw food man seeing a beautiful woman on the street wearing a sexy skirt would barely notice a sight that would make most men at least turn their heads.

Many raw foodists view that change in light of the usual philosophy of deprivation and asceticism. Sex is viewed as "dirty," and the sex drive of average males is viewed as "abnormally high." These raw foodists start to think the rest of the world is wrong, and that eating "stimulating foods" causes this "abnormal" sex drive, which they happen to be liberated from.

Often, the solution to lack of energy and low sex drive is to eat more, especially more "rich" foods. Eat some nuts and seeds. Consuming beans and grains will also cause sex drive to come back, as will animal products. There's not one category of food that is absolutely necessary for sex drive. You just have to consume foods that are a little acid-forming, and not *only* consume fat-free fruits and vegetables. A little sodium intake beyond what's contained in fruits and vegetables will also help restore your sex drive.

As a man, you should start to eat massively to regain your energy and drive. Of course, I'm only talking about healthy, whole foods. But eat. Don't avoid fat, and don't be afraid to make a guacamole with an entire avocado, or eat what you're really craving. If you're exercising, and you're in the "raw freedom" context we've discussed, you'll do just fine.

Lack of Energy

I've met a lot of "tired vegans," and I used to be one of them, although I experienced this symptom on a high-fat raw vegan diet. People complain about feeling exhausted and needing frequent naps to recover.

In vegans, I attribute this mostly to the overconsumption of grains (especially refined grains and flour-based products) and oils, under-consumption of fruit, and under-consumption of total calories.

In raw vegans, it's caused by a high-fat diet combined with the under-consumption of fruit, or by a calorie-restricted diet.

In either case, the solution is to follow a more balanced diet where fats don't predominate, but where you get most of your calories from carbs and a good percentage from fat (15-25% depending on how raw-fruit-heavy your diet is; the higher the fruit content, the lower the fat content should be); and a steady, 10+% protein intake. But the critical factor is calories. Try increasing your daily calorie intake by 500, and see what happens!

Lack of Stamina

Many ex-raw foodists (and sometimes vegans) report that after a few years on a raw vegan diet, they lost the stamina to exercise. For example, in the past they could work out for 60 minutes on the treadmill, and later, until they broke their raw vegan diet, they were finding it hard to do more than 20 minutes, and often needed all day to recover.

I would attribute this in most cases to the same reasons as for lack of energy, but also possibly to a vitamin B12 deficiency.

Constantly Hungry

This symptom is common in vegans but even more so in raw foodists. It's easily explained by the fact that plant foods are not as calorie-dense as animal foods, and also carbohydrates don't satiate as much as protein-based foods.

Vegans and raw foodists need to eat more, but also to satisfy their sweet tooth with fruit, which tends to eliminate most of the cravings by providing the simple carbohydrates the body desperately needs.

When constant hunger is extreme on a low-fat diet, more fat should be added. You can end up constantly hungry if you start exercising a lot and try to get all your calories from unrefined foods. It becomes extremely difficult to get enough calories, so whole food fats come to the rescue. Because you're exercising a lot, you won't have trouble with the weight gain often associated with those foods (I'm talking mainly about nuts, seeds, avocados, and a small amount of unrefined oil).

When I started weight training, as I discussed in chapter XX, I had to increase the fat content in my diet. Otherwise, I was constantly hungry and simply could not satisfy my dietary needs on low-fat foods alone.

Hair Falling Out

This is a symptom that tends to occur mostly in raw vegan women who go on a very low-fat diet or tend to drop weight rapidly. To avoid this, I would encourage an increased consumption of omega 3 rich foods such as flax, walnuts and hemp seeds, and to bring the fat percentage in your diet up above the 15% mark. It can also be a symptom of hypothyroidism, and so is worth getting checked out.

Depression

This is probably the most common serious symptom vegans experience that leads them to change their diet. As we'll see below, it could simply be caused by a vitamin B12 deficiency.

Vitamin B12 Deficiency

This deficiency is common in long-term vegans, but also common in the meat-eating population. Besides severe nervous system degeneration problems, a B12 deficiency can cause fatigue, depression and "brain fog," which could explain why ex-vegans tend to feel instantly better when they start eating meat.

A good supplement is the best way to prevent a B12 deficiency, but perhaps some individuals cannot absorb the supplement optimally, and therefore feel the best results when they get their B12 from animal foods.

Eggs and dairy products are generally a poor source of B12, which would explain why ex-vegans feel so much better when they start eating meat or fish again (just a few ounces of fish provides enough B12 for about two days).

Hypothyroidism

This is a less common symptom that could be caused by a diet rich in raw cruciferous vegetables (like cabbage, broccoli, etc.), which contain thyroid inhibitors known as goitrogens. Consuming a lot of these vegetables is very likely to cause thyroid problems. Unfortunately, these are the same superstar cancer-fighting vegetables with the sulfur compounds.

So, you probably want to include these vegetables in your diet. The simple solution is to steam these vegetables and eat chard, spinach, lettuce, and other non-cruciferous vegetables raw in your salads and smoothies.

Why It's So Hard to Change

I've noticed a certain resistance to change within myself and other people who ate very restricted diets for long periods of time, even when they knew for a fact they needed to make changes in their diet.

When I became a raw foodist back in 1997, I got convinced it was the answer to all humanity's problems. Not only did I think it would bring me to a state of paradise health; I also thought I would never get sick following this diet.

I did not experience paradise health. In fact, my health deteriorated. After many years, I decided to change, but I was still reluctant to make big changes, because I was afraid.

As a raw foodist, you get brainwashed into thinking that cooked foods are really bad for you, that eating any amount of animal product will give you cancer, and that the only foods you could consider cooking would be simple things like asparagus or broccoli.

Even after I realized that a 100% raw food diet was not going to be a lifestyle I would be willing to follow for the rest of my life, I still found myself thinking like a raw foodist.

After a few years on a raw food diet, I experienced serious dental decay directly attributable to the diet. But in spite of this, I was reluctant to completely change my diet.

This was partly because of the weakening of digestion I talked about in chapter X. I was still going through the relative "high" of eating raw, and was perplexed by the dull feelings I experienced after eating cooked foods. For this reason, I still remained convinced at the back of my mind that a pure raw food diet was the ideal diet (except for the fact that it was ruining my teeth), but I had to find an alternative that would be almost as good as what I had been doing.

Most raw foodists and vegans conceive of a sort of imaginary "ladder of evolution" of diets.

At the bottom of the diet would be what is considered the worst diet of all: the SAD diet (Standard American Diet).

Then you have the "health food diet" (eating everything organic and paying attention to food quality), such as what would be promoted by someone like Michael Pollan.

Then we have vegetarianism. Then veganism. Then low-fat, whole foods veganism. Then raw foodism. Then low-fat raw foodism. Then fruitarianism. If you want to reach even higher, you could consider breatharianism!

You could ask yourself instead: "Looking at the available evidence, and evaluating my own life circumstances and personal preferences, what would be the optimal diet I could follow that would be both realistic and super-healthy?"

But that's generally not the path taken by most people.

After a few months or years of raw foodism, many if not most people realize that they won't be able to follow this diet for the rest of their life. They need to find a middle ground. Others experience real health problems, and need to find an alternative.

But reluctance to change makes them go down just one step of the ladder, instead of taking a broader approach. A failing vegan might add a few eggs, but still won't feel ready to eat some fish or meat. A low-fat raw vegan might try to become a low-fat cooked vegan, or something in between.

It's unlikely that diets can really be rated on a scale of health from least healthy to healthiest, at least not in the way we would imagine.

Forget All These Named Diets!

Instead of looking at diets, we should look at *foods*.

What are the foods that you can eat every day? What foods are definitely unhealthy?

What foods do or don't work well in *your* body? Maybe you actually feel great with some good-quality dairy in your diet. Maybe you always get a stomach ache when you eat kale. Maybe you don't like bananas. Then, some foods are clearly unhealthy for anyone. You've read about the problems with high-temperature-cooked meat, and with oxidized vegetable oils, and with overconsumption of omega 6 fatty acids. All sides of the diet spectrum agree that refined sugar and flour are not healthy for anyone. Some foods are very healthy, like vegetables and fruits—but even here, all vegetables contain small amounts of toxins. Some contain goitrogens, some contain oxalates (which block calcium absorption). It is best not to rely on one or two types of vegetable, or one or two food groups, but to diversify. As we've seen, some methods of cooking can be considered healthy, like steaming, sauté, water-stir-frying; some are not, like frying in vegetable oil or barbecuing at high temperatures.

The ladder of healthy diets is just an abstract concept. If you let go of this ladder, and of your self-concept as a "low-fat raw vegan," or whatever you might be, you'll find it easier to let in some change. Trust yourself. You know which foods and preparation methods are healthy. What sounds good? You may find a steamed sweet potato with a side of steamed kale completely delicious and satisfying just like that. One day, you might try some quinoa and discover that, along with some green salad, tomatoes and avocado, it keeps you going all afternoon. Another day, you might have a green smoothie for breakfast just like you always have.

As you become more comfortable trusting yourself and choosing what to eat based on what you feel like eating rather than some restricted rule book of a menu, you may want to set yourself some parameters for when you might eat foods that are *not* part of your regular program. How often would you feel comfortable eating a piece of a cake at a birthday party? Would you eat a burger at a Fourth of July barbecue? Would you ever eat a piece of dark chocolate? Is coconut rice pudding beyond the pale?

Some people have an 80-20 rule. They eat what they know is healthy 80% of the time. They eat foods that they're not actually allergic to, but that they know are unhealthy, 20% of the time. For some, it's 90-10. Some people need to be more black and white.

I've already shared my own approach to making such exceptions. And as I've already said, limiting these exceptions to social occasions is a great idea for at least two reasons:

(1) It means you're not fixing those foods in your own home, which would make it more likely you would eat them more often, and (2) it reflects the intention of having these exceptions at all, which is that they are *exceptions*, often specifically for social reasons, where food is part of the socializing.

You've gotten to the point of acknowledging that you need to make some changes. Congratulations. Now, if you trust your own knowledge and common sense, and listen to your own body and how it reacts to different foods, and if you let go of your identity as a "such-and-such foodist," you'll find yourself effortlessly overcoming the resistance to change.

How to Recover From an Unbalanced Diet

This next part is only meant for people who have been strict or fairly strict raw foodists for an extended period (months or years), have experienced many of the problems I talk about in this book, and also *need* to find balance in their lives again, with a healthy way of eating that is not a 100% raw diet.

The hardest challenge for these people, besides training their digestion to handle a wider variety of foods again, is that *they still think like raw foodists*.

Even after years of no longer eating all-raw, if you followed the raw lifestyle for long enough, there's a good chance *you still think like a raw foodist*. You still, on some level, believe that that a 100% pure raw vegan diet is really the best diet there is, but you are somehow incomplete or flawed for not having been able to make it work. And that perhaps, one day, you'll come back to it. You haven't really accepted that strict raw veganism simply doesn't work for you, and is not good for you.

I see this even in people who had the worst problems on the diet — and especially the ones who were doing everything right, according to the advice given by the gurus. The transition is very slow. For example, one ex-raw foodist who experienced many health problems on a raw vegan diet writes:

> For the most part, I do still feel the fruit-based, plant-based diet is the way to go. And the 100% restrictiveness of it can indeed be beneficial for many, for a time. But the longer I do this, the more I see the shades of grey where I once saw black and white.

In this book I will not propose one way of eating for *everybody*. It's up to you to decide how to incorporate this information.

I can, however, relate my own experience. After years on an all-raw diet, and then years *trying* to be all-raw (most of the time eating mostly fruit and low-fat), I had to conclude that this diet was not good for me. But like the ex-raw foodist I quoted, I still felt that it was the best diet out there. But I felt the strictness of a 100% raw vegan diet wasn't right for me. I was also experiencing some negative symptoms, such as:

- Dental problems
- Disturbed digestion: very loose and watery stools most of the time, and an inability to digest anything but very simple meals, fruits and vegetables, etc.

I didn't like how restricted I felt, and the few negatives physical issues I experienced. But on the other hand, I liked how "light" and "clear" I felt most of the time and the energy I had, and the belief I would not get any serious diseases later in life. Every time I ate cooked foods, I would feel the opposite: dull, guilty, and not "vibrant."

But I also knew that my body needed to transition and get used to a different style of eating. Yet, I still *thought like a raw foodist*. Therefore, I was never really training my body to properly adapt. I would eat all raw and massive amounts of fruit during the day, and then at night I would make a cooked meal. But this meal generally only contained simple things like potatoes, steamed vegetables, and perhaps a little hummus to go with them. I would eat too much, and feel tired and sleepy afterwards.

I would continue this pattern for a while, and then not like the results. So I would revert to 100% raw veganism, thinking I would "get it right this time." I failed, and then reverted to eating cooked foods — but without adapting properly.

Not everybody will be facing the same challenges. Most people have not necessarily been strict raw foodists for long periods, so this advice will not apply to them. Some people already have a fairly balanced program of eating raw and cooked (for example 80% raw with 20% cooked), and are happy about it.

A Word of Advice for Ex-Vegans

I've noticed many people feel that a strict raw vegan diet is no longer appropriate for them. For many, the path of transition away from pure raw foodism starts with eating animal foods. However, many people are still quite affected by both the "raw" and the "vegan" philosophies, and they fail to choose what is best for themselves.

I see a lot of ex-raw foodists mostly focusing on drinking raw milk (sometimes several gallons a week), raw cheese, butter, and eggs. I understand that these foods are less offensive to a former vegan than animal flesh, but current research does not condone eating such large quantities of foods rich in animal-based saturated fats, and very high amounts of cholesterol, in eggs.

A healthier way to eat animal foods would not be agreeable to many former vegans, but nonetheless more recommendable. This would be to avoid dairy for the most part, eat fish (wild or sustainably raised, focusing on fish high in omega 3s), and maybe some occasional organic grass-fed meat, while keeping dairy and eggs to a minimum.

Advice for Recovering Raw Foodists

This next section will not apply to most people, but will be of interest to long-term raw foodists who are desperately trying to find a "way out" of their rigid diet, but have trouble finding it because their body is no longer able to properly digest "normal" foods.

So if you're sick of it and want your health and digestion back, use the advice in this section. Keep in mind that some of these tips are meant to be *temporary*, in order to let your body adapt to a new diet, and in some cases undo some of the damage caused by over-zealous dietary restrictions.

- **Limit the fruit.** It will come across as odd from me to suggest reducing the quantity of fruit you eat because I'm known for being a very pro-fruit person. I want you to look forward to eating a lot of fruit again down the road, but if you need to recover from an overly strict raw food diet and build your digesting potential, limiting your fruit intake is a very important step in the process. Limit yourself to three to four pieces a day. When you've rebuilt your digestion, then you can eat more fruit.

- **Never eat two fruit meals or even snacks in a row.** One of the biggest transition steps I took to go "beyond raw" was to stop eating two large fruit meals in a row. Eat one fruit meal a day, with one fruit snack — max. Your body needs to stop using fruit as a main source of energy. Otherwise, you'll end up eating both large quantities of fruit AND large quantities of starch, which is not advisable. Alternating fruit with other foods will also help you undo some of the damage caused by the high acidity of fruits, such as enamel erosion.

- **Don't just eat large quantities of carbs like potatoes as a meal.** A problem with raw foodists is that whenever they eat cooked foods, they still think "massive." A meal composed of 4 pounds of cooked potatoes is not appropriate, especially when you've been living on a raw food diet for a while. You'll feel sleepy. Instead, balance your meal with a variety of foods: starch, salad, vegetables, protein, a little avocado, etc.

- **Don't expect to feel great at first. It will take time to adapt.** Going from a cooked food diet to a raw food diet is a big change, and you probably remember feeling terrible at first as your body adapted to the next diet. Introducing cooked foods after a long period not eating it can also feel that way. So give your body time, and don't expect everything to be back in order in a matter of days.

- **Don't give up on any food you want to eat.** It's easy for raw foodists to automatically assume that because they can't immediately digest a food, it is bad for them. Sometimes, it's all in the mind too. We eat something the night before, and feel bad the next day. And, we think the two events are related. But sometimes, the events are not related. Maybe you feel bad because of something else, and you're blaming the food for it. If there's a food you really want to be able to eat and tolerate, give yourself some time. Try it again, after a few weeks. And then, try it again after month or two. Eventually, you will be able to digest all healthy foods.

- **Admit that you need to find balance.** This is probably the biggest step you can take. It's important to admit to yourself that going from one extreme to the next is not going to solve all your health problems. Avoid the temptation to jump into the next diet, such as "Paleo" or do endless "diet shopping," and rely on your common sense. You will probably never have a completely normal and effortless relationship with food (like most people), but it's important to find a balance, and avoid extremes such as the constant need to "detox" and punish yourself for your past sins.

- **Eat a small amount of cooked food, every day** — You may need to train your body to eat cooked foods after a long period of abstinence. The key to this process is starting slowly, and building up. Don't go to a Chinese buffet on your first day! Start with simple foods, like cooked sweet potatoes and vegetables, in reasonable quantities, and add new foods and slightly larger quantities every day.

- **Train your body to consume protein.** This is a bit counterintuitive, but as mentioned earlier in this book, eating foods that are concentrated in protein can help your digestion. In a vegetarian diet, beans and nuts would not be enough to have that effect. I would suggest using some "fake meats" such as soy products for a period of time. I know these foods are not necessarily the healthiest, but they will serve the purpose of rebuilding your digestion. Start slowly! Of course, lean meat and fish, in small quantities, will work great. Eggs are more high-fat foods than high-protein foods, as is cheese, and most dairy.

- **Consume a small amount of salt every day.** Eliminating salt completely will make it difficult if not impossible to find complete "freedom" in your diet to be able to occasionally eat out and so on. So having a small quantity of salt with your food every day will avoid this problem.

Top Mistakes Made By Raw Foodists Whenever They Eat Cooked Foods or Go Back To a Cooked Food Approach

- **They blame the food for their body's reactivity.** After however long eating such a restricted diet, a raw foodist's body is quite reactive when presented with a food outside of that small palette. They decide to eat a few lightly toasted nuts. When their nose runs a bit, they think about oxidized fats and evaporated vitamins and acrylamide and every other scrap of data they've picked up about cooked food as toxic. Until a recovering raw foodist has really habituated herself and her body to eating cooked food, she'll be so accustomed to thinking like a raw foodist that she'll be *looking* for symptoms when she eats cooked food and may even bring them on herself!

- **They eat cooked starch *after* eating a lot of fruit.** Low-fat raw is fruit; low-fat cooked is starch, right? So, too often, a recovering raw foodist will try to cover both bases. Thinking like a raw foodist, he'll eat his fill of fruit in the large quantities to which he's accustomed. Then, he'll move on to his potatoes or quinoa. This is a whole lot of carbohydrate of two different kinds, one on top of the other. *Anyone* would feel uncomfortable after eating that amount, not just a raw foodist trying to retrain his gut!

- **The "timid" version—they eat just steamed veggies.** The recovering raw foodist has heard about goitrogens in cruciferous vegetables like broccoli, cauliflower, kale, mustard, arugula and the list goes on, and oxalates in vegetables like chard, spinach, beets, quinoa, amaranth…and has become truly afraid to eat them raw, but also afraid to leave them out completely because of their great benefits. She has also heard that steaming is the healthiest way to cook, because it depletes nutrients the least. She's afraid of baking potatoes because of the dry heat, and isn't sure about steaming them. She doesn't really remember how to cook grains and is worried about the phytates anyway. So, she end up subsisting almost entirely on steamed vegetables—she's kind of worried about the

231

sugar in fruit, and of course she doesn't do well with fat. She gets dopey and confused, has trouble concentrating, her hair starts to fall out…She has night-time encounters with the almond butter jar and secret shame-trips to the gluten free bakery. Part of the point of embracing cooked foods again is to have *more* options, both nutritionally and socially, not less! Don't get drowned in the minutiae!

• **"The kitchen is always open"—they overeat massively.** Some people just seem to have a strong constitution. They eat so much food, and then not long after, they're eating again, a completely different kind of food, and again, in large quantities. (This sounds like a stereotypical "guy" thing, but I've met plenty of women who are that way too.) This is the kind of person especially whose appetite will be triggered when transitioning away from just raw foods. So many options! Big banana smoothie for breakfast, baked good with mid-morning coffee (yes, coffee!), Indian all you can eat buffet for lunch, potato chips and M&Ms in the break room, big bowl of rice and beans with some cheese on top, popcorn with an evening-at-home movie. Aside from the fact that this will eventually cause weight gain unless a person is physically active to match such huge consumption, it is very hard on the body to have to process food in that quantity. In fact, most people's bodies won't let them do this indefinitely. They will get sick or otherwise uncomfortable, and will have to come back into balance.

These are the main mistakes people make when transitioning toward a more permissive diet. As you look at them, you can probably see yourself in one or the other. So, you know what your own tendencies are, and can bear this in mind as you make your transition so that you can avoid these pitfalls.

Answering the Critics

In the past you recommended a low-fat diet. Have you changed your mind?

In the past, I recommended raw foodists stick to a higher-fruit diet rather than a lower-fruit diet. That's because on a raw food diet, calories can either come from fat or simple sugar. There is no in-between, because the raw food diet doesn't contain a lot of protein, and because no complex carbs are consumed. In this context, sticking to a low-fat diet increases insulin sensitivity and enables one to process the necessary calories coming from high amounts of fruit in the diet. This pattern of eating makes a lot more sense than the alternative, which is to base your diet on nuts and seeds, with vegetables.

The percentage of fat that is considered healthy varies from one author to the next. Dr. Doug Graham, essentially the initiator of this way of eating in the raw food world, recommends 10% or less of total calories coming from fat. 10% is the upper limit, not the target. In practice, that means half an avocado to one avocado a day for most people, but often less if fewer calories are consumed.

In practice, I always tended to eat 15% of total calories from fat on a high-raw or all-raw diet. I found 10% of total calories a little difficult to follow and felt more balanced on 15% fat.

But in this book, we're not discussing an all-raw diet. We're discussing a *raw freedom plan* that can be followed by people who have some interest in the raw food lifestyle but don't want to do it 100% — and in some cases don't want to do it at all.

The percentage of fat you consume is something you can experiment with. I still recommend a rather low-fat diet, but I'm willing to go as high as 25% as long as not too much sugar is consumed (including fruit).

Fat content in your diet has to match activity levels. Active and athletic people can eat more fat. But again, the more fruit you eat in your diet, the less fat you should eat. That's because the combination of loads of simple sugar and fat can be problematic.

Ironman athlete and vegan author Brendan Brazier also recommends a higher fat intake for more active people. He discusses this in detail in his book *Thrive*, and also lays it out in his article in VegKitchen.com: "A very low-fat diet is ok for a low to moderately active person. However, a highly active person, especially an endurance athlete who has adopted a plant-based diet, will benefit by adding good quality fats to his/her meals."[11]

The bottom line is I still recommend a low-fat diet compared to the amount consumed by most people (40+%). However, a super-low-fat diet (less than 10% of total calories) is not a health requirement for most people. If fat calories are coming from healthy sources (whole foods, such as nuts and seeds, and foods rich in omega 3 fats), and one is not consuming most calories from simple sugars in fruit, then a higher percentage of fat is not going to impair your health.

Do you still consider yourself a raw foodist?

I've never actually considered myself a "raw foodist" since I stopped eating 100% raw. You wouldn't call someone a "vegetarian" if they ate a small amount of meat every day, or every week.

---

11   http://www.vegkitchen.com/nutrition/vegan-athlete/

Should your previous books be burned in a big bonfire?

I stand by what I wrote in my old books, but of course with time a few things change and you come to different conclusions on smaller details. If someone wants to follow a raw food diet or a high-raw diet, the best way to do it is by following the plan I laid out in my books. *Raw Freedom* is for people who want to incorporate the best of both worlds — raw and cooked — in a sensible plan, when the restrictions of a raw food diet simply didn't work.

You sell books on the raw food diet, isn't that a contradiction?

When I wrote my first book on the raw food diet in 1999 (*Sunfood Cuisine*), I was filled with enthusiasm about this way of life. I was just 23.

In the space of a few years, I accumulated a lot of knowledge on the raw food diet by reading approximately one hundred books on the subject, and spending about three years traveling the US and meeting influential raw foodists.

I told my stories in my most recent book, *Raw Food Controversies*, which some people have called my "raw food autobiography," although a big part of the book covers important research on the topic of raw vegan nutrition.

I have written many raw food books, but all of them are different than the average raw food book. My first "theory" book, *The Raw Secrets*, was the first published book, to my knowledge, that presented a critique of the raw food diet from the point of view of someone who was a raw foodist and had experienced a health decline after following the diet.

In my first book, I came from a much more *natural hygiene* background, and my main criticism was of the high-fat raw food diet (based on vegetables, oils, and insane quantities of nuts, seeds, and avocados), which I felt was making most raw foodists sick. My criticism still stands, and everything I wrote on the topic remains absolutely accurate.

In many of my books, I promoted a low-fat, high-fruit raw food diet as an alternative to the high-fat raw food diet that was making people sick. I still think that a low-fat raw food diet is a much superior program to the "standard" raw food diet promoted almost everywhere.

Nowhere in my books did I claim I ate a 100% raw food diet, except perhaps in my very early writings from the late 90s when I was actually doing it. Since then, I made it absolutely clear that I was not and did not intend to be seen as a 100% raw foodist.

I'm still interested in making raw foods the main part of my diet, but I don't consider myself a raw foodist, and it's pretty clear if you actually read my books that I have not claimed to be one for a long time.

I published *The Raw Secrets* when I was just 26. At the time, I felt I had accomplished something major and helped a lot of people reevaluate their diet and improve their health.

Of course, if you go back over ten years, to my early books like *The Raw Secrets*, there are some issues on which I have changed my mind.

Eating for Weight Loss...or Gain

Tips for Weight Gain or Body-Building Nutrition

This topic is rarely discussed, because most people who show an interest in raw foods are motivated to follow the diet to lose weight. Individuals needing to *gain* weight, either from being underweight or because they desire to gain muscle mass, are left in the dark.

Let's cover gaining muscle mass, because that's what nearly all underweight individuals primarily lack.

Gaining muscle is a very simple yet challenging process that can be summarized with the following equation:

An intense weightlifting regimen + Eating enough calories to allow for growth (in addition to getting enough sleep)

People who engage in weightlifting and yet fail to gain noticeable muscle mass are either not eating enough, or not training hard enough. In some cases, they may be training too hard, and not allowing their bodies to recuperate.

Although I've had some interest in weightlifting in the past, I've never really managed to gain a significant amount of muscle mass until recently. I was more of a runner. But in late October 2012, I started a serious and consistent weight-training program. I managed to add almost 15 pounds to my frame in about 4 months, while keeping the same relative body fat level. There's been a marked change in my body that everybody who knows me has noticed.

The weight-training program I followed was designed by a trainer I hired. I started with a three-day-a-week full-body training with machines, then moved on to free weights. I then switched to a four-day-a week routine, each day focusing on completely different muscle groups. Each workout takes between 60 and 90 minutes, including warm-up.

When I started weight training, I became very hungry. Much more so than when I was running consistently in the past. And I knew that muscle gain was not possible without a "massive eating plan" to accompany it. So I followed my hunger and ate the necessary amounts.

Having tried a similar approach in the past while following a mainly raw food diet, I immediately noticed quicker results on my current program. While I do believe I could have built muscle on a 100% raw food diet, I'm convinced it would have been much more difficult. I noticed the difference in in my strength gains, reaching personal bests in every single category of lifting.

I simply allowed myself to eat a lot of food, and not worry about the raw percentage. I added one scoop of raw protein powder (I used either the "Sunwarrior" or the "Growing Naturals" brand) in my morning and post-workout smoothies. My morning green smoothie was essentially the same and I did not consume more than 500 or 600 calories for breakfast. I allowed myself to eat more fat than I normally would, in order to get the necessary calories. That usually meant I ate an entire avocado for lunch, along with other foods, such as salad, cooked sweet potatoes, beans, and tofu. I often ate an entire avocado for dinner as well. I found myself consuming fish more frequently (usually wild salmon or rare tuna steaks), but otherwise stuck to a plant-based diet. I rarely ate eggs (but sometimes did), and tried to load up on fruit whenever hungry. The biggest difference was that I ate bigger quantities and did not worry as much about the fat, and also that my diet was not nearly as raw as before.

I believe that in this case, lowering the raw food percentage in the diet helps, because as we've seen, calories in raw foods are less accessible. It can become particularly challenging to consume enough raw foods to allow for muscle growth. I know some people may disagree with me and say "all you gotta do is eat the food," but I simply haven't met anybody who obtained the results I did, which is essentially a complete body makeover, in such a short period of time on a raw food diet.

I did not take any drugs, creatine, or other artificial preparations. However, sometimes, in order to get through a particularly tough workout, I did consume drinks containing refined sugar (Gatorade) when I forgot to bring my own recovery drink with me. I actually did not worry too much about sugar or carb consumption on my workout days, especially after a workout. My recovery drink, consumed right after the workout, contained at least 250 calories (more like 300) of carbs, usually from fruit, mixed with a raw protein powder.

I did start to experiment with vegan athlete Brendan Brazier's "Pre-Workout Energizer" formula, which contains, among other plant extracts, green tea and yerba mate. The results using this product were particularly good, and I did not find that this moderate caffeine consumption negatively affected me otherwise.

So that's my experience. As I'm writing this book, I'm still on a weight-training program that I intend to follow through the summer, to see where I can go. But after that, I don't know if I'll keep it up in the same fashion. I miss the high that running gives me, so it's possible that I'll switch to a program that emphasizes running, with a few days of weight training. In this case, I'll change my nutrition accordingly to be more carb-heavy, with less fat.

My advice for people (usually men) who desire to gain weight, ideally muscle mass, is to follow a similar approach. You'll get best results if you hire a personal trainer to design a program for you. But the program is only one part of the answer. Nutrition is equally important. For those wanting to gain muscle mass who are already making the necessary efforts at the gym, my advice is to:

- Lower the percentage of raw foods in the diet to allow for more calorie-dense foods to take their place.

- On training days, don't worry so much about "empty calories" such as drinks that might contain sugar, fruit juice; or white rice or flour.

- Eat a lot of food! That's the main advice. You should be feeling hungry and devouring big meals regularly.

- Increase the fat content of your diet (in the form of healthy fat such as avocado, nuts, and seeds), and in this context, a little unrefined, unheated oil like olive oil is certainly okay.

- Vegan products such as the raw sprouted rice protein powders made by Sunwarrior or Growing Naturals can be excellent tools in rounding out your nutrition. Also check out the Vega brand of products by Brendan Brazier.

- You can do this program on a vegan diet or not. Make sure to consume plenty of beans, unrefined carbs (such as root vegetables), fruits, and vegetables. In the animal protein department, lean proteins such as fish or grass-fed meat will give you the best results.

Eating for Weight Loss

Unsurprisingly, my advice for weight loss is basically the opposite of the advice for muscle- or weight gain.

It is not necessary to eat a raw food diet to lose weight, but it's necessary to make drastic changes in the calorie-nutrient ratio of your food. That means: something's gotta go.

Some people get good results by restricting carbs, increasing protein, and maintaining a good fat intake. That's the traditional diet advice, in many forms.

I personally think the best approach is still to restrict or almost eliminate fat (temporarily), as well as eliminating all sources of refined carbohydrates (including bread, sugar, pastries, and anything containing flour). Coconuts, avocados, nuts, and seeds should be eliminated (temporarily) or restricted.

My own mom followed this approach and lost 60 pounds, without gaining it back. The diet also did wonders for other aspects of her health. She lived mainly on oatmeal, brown rice, vegetable soups, salads, bean dishes, vegetables, and some fruit. This is essentially the approach championed by Dr. Esselstyn and Dr. McDougall.

Another approach is to eat more raw foods. As we've seen, raw foods are less dense in calories than cooked foods, and the calories they contain are less accessible. The only exception would be some fat sources, such as any oil (olive oil included). Avocados, coconut milk, and some nuts can be fattening. However, almonds are okay, because of their high fiber content.

So if you have a good amount of weight to lose, find the ratio of raw foods that is appropriate for you, but err on the side of "more raw food." The alternative is to follow a program similar to the one I gave my mom to lose that weight. In any case, you'll be reducing fat, and eating only whole plant foods. However, on the raw food program, more fat is allowed, because raw foods in general are not as calorie-dense. Essentially, following the program I presented in my other books will take you to the results you desire.

Appendix 1

Glossary of Raw Food Terms

Acrylamide—the toxic byproduct created when **starches** are fried at high heat. Often the first piece of evidence that converts people to Raw foods.

Appetite—a hankering to eat something; usually something quite specific. Contrasted with **Hunger**, below.

Blender—probably the most important piece of equipment in a **raw foodist's** kitchen aside from a sharp knife and cutting board! **Blenders** are used mainly for liquid foods, like smoothies or salad dressings. They break down fibers, and homogenize everything. **Blenders** can cost just a few dollars at a thrift store, or you can go all the way up over $400 for a workhorse like the Vita-Mix or Blendtec. No need to do this as a newbie, though.

Calorie Dense—describes food that contains a large amount of calories per weight. For example, 100 grams of fresh figs contains just 74 calories, but 100 grams of dried figs contains 249 calories. The dried figs are more **calorie dense** than the fresh ones. See **Nutrient Dense** below.

Carbohydrate—the most important **Macronutrient** we consume. **Carbohydrates** may be simple (**Sugars**, see below) or complex (**Starches**, see below).

Dehydrator—like an oven, with a heating element and fan, but only heats foods between approximately 85-165 degrees Fahrenheit. **Dehydrators** have been used for years to dry out fruits, vegetables, herbs, and even smoked meats, for long-term shelf-stable storage. Gourmet **raw foodists** have repurposed the dehydrator to take the place of an oven in cooked foods, and create complex dishes that mimic the density of cooked foods without having been subjected to high heat.

Diet—a way of eating that is followed for at least 80% of the time, life-long. It is not just some quick fix to lose or gain weight. **Diet** is one of the key pillars of a healthy lifestyle. See **Natural Hygiene**, below.

Exercise—another crucial aspect of a healthy lifestyle. **Exercise** means moving the body, preferably out of doors, challenging it to get stronger and more capable, preferably in a way that feels enjoyable to the person. See **Natural Hygiene**, below.

Fasting—complete abstinence from all nutritive substance (a small amount of water is allowed). True fasting does not include drinking juice or some concoction of lemon and cayenne pepper with refined sweetener. Water-**fasting** is the first recommended action in any illness. Regular short fasts are also encouraged for maintenance.

Fat—refers to adipose tissue in the body, but also to the **Macronutrient** most commonly overeaten and most likely to cause problems.

Fatty Foods—in the context of the raw diet, fatty foods include avocados, olives, nuts, seeds, cacao, durian to some extent, and all oils (coconut, olive, flaxseed, hemp, etc.).

Food—what we eat to sustain life.

Food-Combining—a set of rules formulated by early **Natural Hygiene** teachers and designed to prevent the simultaneous presence in the stomach of foods requiring an acid environment for digestion, like **fats** and **proteins**, and foods requiring an alkaline environment for digestion, like **starches**. The scientific status of these rules is controversial, but in practical terms they are definitely useful guidelines for a person trying to simplify their diet.

Food Processor—chops, grinds, mixes foods, especially vegetables, nuts, and dried fruit. Whereas the **blender** makes liquid concoctions, the **food processor** is mostly used for pâtés, pestos, salsas, and nut-date-type treats. A food processor usually also has attachments for chopping and shredding vegetables. There are some manual tools that cut vegetables into interesting shapes too, like mandolins and spiralizers.

Fruit—in the context of raw food diets, fruit generally refers to sweet fruits. Avocados, tomatoes, bell peppers, zucchini, etc., which are fruits botanically speaking, are considered vegetables (or a fat, in the case of avocado).

Fruitarian—a person who eats all, or at least 80%, of their diet as fruit. Fruitarians will generally include in their definitions all kinds of fruit, including avocados, tomatoes, bell peppers, and other vegetables that are botanically fruits.

Guru—someone who claims to know all about a diet or lifestyle and who lectures authoritatively and insistently, and often attracts a fanatical following. Beware of gurus!

Health—a state of optimal balance in the holistic sense—body, mind, and spirit, whereby an individual can achieve his or her maximum potential. This will vary from individual to individual because of genetic or environmental factors, but can be supported or improved by attention to **Diet** and lifestyle. Outward signs of health include clear skin, absence of breath- or body-odor, a good level of physical fitness and stamina, and a generally calm, optimistic, peaceful outlook on life. See **Natural Hygiene**, below.

High-fat diet—a diet in which more than 20% of calories come from **Fat**. The modern gourmet raw diet, which mimics familiar cooked foods with elaborate recipes, is by definition a high-fat diet, with its reliance on nuts, seeds, oils and a few very low-calorie vegetables. Some poorly planned early versions of the **raw food** diet from a **Natural Hygiene** approach also ended up very high in **Fat** due to inadequate **Fruit** and overuse of nuts.

Hunger—in contrast with **Appetite**, the genuine physical sensation that the stomach is empty and requires food.

Juicing—the extraction of the liquid part of a fruit or vegetable; often a combination of fruits and vegetables are prepared together. Many health-oriented authors advocate **juicing** as a good way to "mainline" the vitamins and minerals without the fibrous portion; however, fruit juices and the juices of vegetables like carrots and beets are far too high in sugar unbuffered by the fiber, and leafy vegetables contain small amounts of toxins that get concentrated by removal of the fiber. Some people think that it's not necessarily desirable to "mainline" vitamins and minerals, but it's also worth considering that this is a relatively easy way to obtain some of the nutrients we so need in our modern lifestyles.

Living Foods—like **raw foods,** the term **living foods** refers to plant foods in their natural state. The difference is that **living foods** places emphasis on the presence of *life force* in the food, including cultures in fermented foods like sauerkraut; or **sprouts**, which are growing right up until you eat them. Some cooked foods, like miso, can be considered **living foods** because they contain live cultures. This version of the **raw food** diet does not include dried, dehydrated or frozen foods.

Low-fat diet—in the context of the **Natural Hygiene** approach to **Raw Foods**, a low-fat diet is a diet containing not more than 20% of *calories* (not volume) from fat; many authorities recommend no more than 10%. The optimal percentage of fat will vary from person to person but generally speaking, the higher the percentage of simple sugars in the diet (including from fruit), the lower the percentage of fat should be.

Macronutrient—refers to the three calorie-containing components of food: **Carbohydrate, Fat,** and **Protein.** People tend to worry too much about the second two.

Micronutrient—factors like vitamins, minerals and phytochemicals present in tiny quantities in the food we eat or absorbed from the environment; necessary to the proper functioning of our bodies. Everyone, no matter their diet, should pay attention to Vitamin B12,

Vitamin D, and perhaps the omega 3s DHA and EPA; otherwise, if you get enough calories, your bases should be covered.

Natural Hygiene—one of the oldest approaches to raw food eating. **Natural hygiene** teaches an old-fashioned approach to a healthy lifestyle in harmony with nature. **Diet** is only one aspect of the lifestyle, which also includes avoidance of environmental toxins both literal and metaphorical, spending time outside, plenty of quality **Rest**, and **Exercise**. Foods are eaten in their natural state as much as possible, although cooking of grains and starchy vegetables and creating simple dressings for salads is permitted. The use of **Food as Medicine** is explicitly discouraged. **Fasting** is recommended as the first line of action when experiencing any ailment.

Nutrient Dense—describes food that contains a large amount of **micronutrients** per weight. For example, 100 grams of kale contains significant amounts of vitamins A, C, and K, and Calcium, Magnesium, Phosphorus, Potassium, and Sodium, but 100 grams of cooked white rice only contains tiny amounts of certain B vitamins, and small amounts of Magnesium, Potassium, Phosphorus, and Manganese. Kale is more **nutrient dense** than white rice. Note that when comparing different versions of the same food in its raw state versus cooked or dried, the dried or cooked versions may be more nutrient dense than the raw version, because the moisture is removed, making it more dense per weight. See **calorie dense,** above.

Protein—a **macronutrient** obtained from food, together with **fat** and **carbohydrate**. **Protein** is essential for muscle growth, and people tend to worry far too much about getting enough of it. Maintenance protein requirements for adults are in fact rather small. If a person on a **raw food** diet eats adequately for their size and activity level, protein should not be an issue. On the other hand, protein is very useful in retraining a digestive system weakened by too much time on an overly restrictive diet.

Raw foods—foods that have not been heated above the temperature at which a seed will sprout—as low as 98 degrees Fahrenheit or as high as 120 degrees, depending who you ask. This may include dehydrated fruits and nuts, expensive dehydrated 'superfood' powders, and dehydrated prepared raw dishes. In the **low-fat**, **natural hygiene** sense, and for large numbers of raw foodists outside of the big urban centers in the US and Europe, **raw foods** instead refers to whole, uncooked fruits and vegetables in their natural state, or close to it. These foods are generally to be eaten unprocessed—no extracted oils, although small amounts of nut butters from whole nuts or seeds are OK; **juicing** is generally discouraged, although smoothies made from whole fruits and vegetables, blended right before consumption, are fine; no honey, agave, or other processed sweeteners—why bother, when you have dates? **Note:** "**raw foods**" generally refers to plant foods—fruits, vegetables, seeds. However, there are people who eat raw animal products also, such as raw dairy products, raw eggs; even raw meat (sushi and steak tartare taken further!). But when you hear **"Raw foods"** or **"Raw foodist,"** you should expect the vast majority of the time to be hearing about plant foods and vegans.

Raw foodist—a person who consumes most or all of their diet uncooked. This can mean food not heated above a certain temperature but possibly quite refined or processed, or it can mean a person who eats primarily raw and minimally processed fresh fruits and vegetables. It may refer to a person who eats **raw foods** including raw animal products, but this is by far the exception. See **Raw foods** above.

Rest—a key component of **Health** according to **Natural Hygiene**. Rest means adequate sleep but also avoidance of overwork and stress; the inclusion of some downtime or playtime in one's life.

Sprouting—germinating seeds to produce baby plants, or to render nuts and seeds more digestible. **Living Foods** strongly advocates baby greens and sprouts as extremely **nutrient dense**, but this author discourages their use, as they are barely more **nutrient dense** than mature greens, and they contain far more toxins. It is also not desirable to make nuts more digestible, as it is important to eat them only in small quantities.

Starches—complex **carbohydrates** composed of strings of sugars. Starches include vegetables such as potatoes, sweet potatoes, yams, beets, winter squash, and all grains, gluten-containing and otherwise, as well as the pseudograins—amaranth, quinoa, buckwheat.

Sugar—simple **carbohydrates** composed of one or two molecules. In the context of a **raw food diet**, simple sugars come from whole, ripe fruits. Cooking of **starchy** vegetables like sweet potatoes, or grains like rice, breaks down the starch and yields simple sugars, which is why they are easier to digest that way. The version of the raw food diet presented here does not include simple sugars in the form of agave nectar or honey as sometimes used by raw foodists.

Superfoods—processed at low temperatures and ground into powders, and sold at great expense, these are foods claimed to contain more than normal amounts of vitamins, minerals, hormones, and you name it. Better to spend your money on whole, fresh foods.

Vegan—refers to a person or a diet that abstains from animal products of all kinds: meat, eggs, dairy; also usually honey. As shorthand, the standard **Raw food** diet gets called a Raw vegan diet; however, the word **Vegan** carries a lot more implications than simply "plant-based." It involves an ethical component; the desire not to harm animals or take any of their products from them, so that ethical vegans also do not wear leather, etc. Many raw foodists use honey, and generally haven't thought so much about this aspect of avoiding animal products.

Appendix 2

How can you tell if you're orthorexic?

Give yourself a point for each question. The more points you accumulate, the more "orthorexic" you are:

#1: Do you spend more than three hours a day thinking about healthy food? If you do, give yourself a point; if you spend more time, give yourself two points.

#2: Do you plan tomorrow's food today? So, do you think "What am I going to eat tomorrow?"

#3: Do you care more about the virtue of what you eat than the pleasure you get from eating it?

#4: Have you found that as the quality of your diet has improved, the quality of your life has diminished?

#5: Do you keep getting stricter with yourself?

#6: Do you sacrifice experiences you once enjoyed to eat the foods you believe are right?

#7: Do you feel a sense of self-esteem when you eat healthy food; do you look down on others who don't?

#8: Do you feel guilt or self-loathing when you stray from your diet?

#9: Does your diet socially isolate you?

#10: When you are eating the way think you are supposed to, do you feel a peaceful sense of total control?

When I look at the questionnaire above, I can honestly say there was a point in my life where I would have answered "yes" to almost every single question.

I used to think about food all the time, to the point that it would be my main topic of conversation with EVERYONE. I tried all kinds of strict "detox" diets, hoping to finally experience the benefits promised to me by the raw food gurus, but nothing worked.

In fact, with time, I became sicker and sicker. I was so obsessed with this ideal of raw foodism, but at the same time so unsatisfied and filled with cravings, to the point that I was having dreams of eating cooked junk foods. In one dream, I was eating a giant chocolate cake, and woke up the next morning feeling so guilty, as if I had just killed somebody.

Nowadays, I still think it's important to have some measure of control over your diet but I don't think anyone should be so obsessed that their decisions are driven by an ideal rather than by common sense. For example:

#1: Don't eat anything and everything just because it's "raw."

#2: Don't refuse to eat something that's not organic, IF the alternative food is less healthy.

#3: Don't think that just because you value healthful living everyone else should feel the same way, or that you're somehow better and more "enlightened" than they are. This just alienates your friends and family.

#4: Compare yourself with yourself, rather than with others, such as raw food "gurus."

#5: Realize that it's okay to give yourself goals, but sometimes fall off the wagon and pick yourself up again. It's just part of the process.

#6: Stay a bit flexible in your approach, and be open to new ideas. You will never learn anything new with a closed mind.

#7: Treat others and yourself with dignity and respect. Food is only one aspect of your life.

Appendix 3

Recipes

If you are a jaded raw foodist, you probably know lots of recipes already. If you're raw-curious but haven't made a go of it, you've probably tried all kinds of recipes too. Either way, you're not coming to this book primarily for recipes.

And a big point I've wanted to make throughout this book is: *you don't need a ton of recipes to make this diet work!*

Making a simple green salad while your sweet potatoes are steaming, and eating them together, isn't something that even requires instructions. Hummus with a medley of steamed and fresh vegetables for dipping can be a delightful meal. You can use canned beans in your salads and to make your hummus unless/until you decide to soak beans in big batches and then freeze them divided into two-cup amounts equivalent to one can. Things like rice and quinoa generally have cooking instructions on the package, or if you have a rice cooker, it will have the water to grain ratio posted on the side and will do all the work for you.

In this simple, intuitive, flowing setting, spices and condiments are really yours to figure out rather than something a recipe should tell you by the half teaspoon of this and pinch of that. Start small, and see for yourself if you like oregano with your tomatoes, or ginger with your cauliflower.

With all that said, here are some recipes, an eclectic mix of things I have enjoyed. Some of these are my own creations; some were contributed by my friends and associates.

Let's start with **Smoothies**, since they play such a big part in a low-fat raw diet and are such a good component of any diet.

Generally, these smoothies will serve 1-2 people, depending on appetite and activity level, but they are also very easy to scale up or down.

Smoothies

Fred's Green Smoothie

1 cup almond milk (store-bought, low-fat, oil-free)

½ cup frozen blueberries

1 pear, diced

1-2 bananas

As many handfuls of spinach as you feel like fitting in the blender

1 scoop raw protein powder (optional)

Put all in the blender in the order listed, and blend until smooth and uniform in color.

Green Revolution Smoothie

1 cup water (or more if needed)

4 medium bananas

1 handful chard leaves

5-6 small-to-medium leaves or **2-3** big leaves black (dinosaur) kale

Blend water with bananas first; add greens progressively, and blend until smooth.

Lee's Pinky Green Smoothie

Water (as necessary)

1 pint strawberries

3 medium bananas

2 handfuls spinach

Blend, admire, eat...

A Winning Green Smoothie

2 cups papaya, diced

5-6 medium dates (or 2-3 medjool dates)

2 frozen bananas

1 handful parsley

Water, as needed

Blend all ingredients together. Use a little water if needed to achieve the desired consistency.

Kale Lover's Green Smoothie

3 bananas

2 apples (golden or other sweet variety)

1 cup water

1 ½ cups kale or mixed baby greens**

** "Mixed baby greens" is a mix of various young greens. It can be found in most produce stores and health food stores. The best types are the organic brands.

Blend the bananas, apples and water. Add in the kale or mixed baby greens and continue blending until smooth.

The Workout Green Smoothie

2 cups water

3 bananas

1 cup blueberries (fresh or frozen)

3-4 large stalks celery

Blend water with bananas and blueberries. Add in the celery stalks, and blend until smooth. This is a great drink after your morning exercise. It's juicy enough, and provides natural sugars from the fruit, and sodium from the celery.

Banana Slug Green Smoothie

1 cup water

3 bananas

2 pears

2 cups romaine lettuce

Blend everything. If you think lettuce and bananas can't combine, think again!

Best Fruit Smoothie Ever

3 cups mango

1½ cup papaya (or fresh or frozen berries of your choice)

1 to 2 cups greens of your choice (optional)

Blend all ingredients with enough water to reach desired consistency. For a light green smoothie, add in 1 or 2 cups of greens such as parsley, spinach or lettuce.

Dressings

Now, let's move on to dressings. These are quite versatile, which makes them central to this way of eating. They can be eaten on a salad, or over steamed vegetables. They can be blended with cooled cooked beans to make a dip that is satisfying and protein-rich without being overly fatty (like hummus but using different beans). The **creamy kelp dressing,** the **ginger dressing,** and the **ranch dressing** would be particularly good blended with beans and made into dips. The dressings are also *very* easy to make!

Creamy Kelp Dressing

1½ cup tomatoes

1 tablespoon agave nectar

1½ tablespoons flavored balsamic vinegar*

3 tablespoons tahini or almond butter

1 tablespoon kelp powder or granules

5-6 chopped chives

Blend all ingredients.

*May be replaced by regular balsamic vinegar, or lime juice. Flavored balsamic vinegar can be found in many health food stores; it may be flavored with blackberries, cherries, or other fruits—your choice!

Tomato Basil Dressing

1 pound ripe plum tomatoes, chopped

2 garlic cloves, crushed

1/2 cup basil leaves

1/4 teaspoon sea salt

1 tablespoon extra-virgin olive oil

Put the extra virgin olive oil in a bowl and add the chopped tomatoes and crushed garlic. Tear up the basil and add to the bowl. Sprinkle the sea salt on top. Let this sit out on the counter or table for at least 3 hours. The sea salt will start to break down the juices of the tomatoes as it marinates. The longer it marinates, the better.

Transfer all into a food processor and blend. This tomato-basil dressing is especially good over a salad of shredded zucchini, mushrooms, and onion.

Ginger Oriental Dressing

2 teaspoons ginger root, freshly grated

1 to 2 cloves fresh garlic, minced

4 tablespoons Braggs Liquid Aminos or Soy Sauce

4 tablespoons Water

4 teaspoons orange juice

2 teaspoons white vinegar

Blend all ingredients. Good with cabbage and carrot salads.

Ginger Dressing

1 medium carrot

2 tablespoon onion

1/3 cup oil

1/3 **cup** water

1 **tablespoon** honey

½ **tablespoon** tamari

2 – 3 **inches** fresh ginger

2 **tablespoons** Apple Cider Vinegar

Dash cayenne

Blend, and enjoy over salad or steamed vegetables.

Avo-Mango Delight

1 **medium** avocado

1 **medium** mango

¼ **cup** water

Blend 1/4 cup of water with avocado and mango. Serve over salad.

Avocado Basil Dressing

½ **medium** avocado

¼ **cup** water

4 **medium** fresh basil leaves

1 **tablespoon** fresh lemon juice

celery powder, kelp or dulse **to taste**

Blend avocado and water until smooth. Then add basil until it shows in flecks of green but is not fully blended.

Peppery Tart Papaya Dressing

2-3 cups medium papaya (about 1 Hawaiian papaya)

1 cup avocado (about one medium)

¼ cup lemon juice

1 tablespoon apple cider vinegar

2 tablespoons fresh basil, chiffonade

Pinch sea salt (**to taste**)

Optional: 1 tablespoon extra-virgin olive oil

Optional: 2 tablespoons papaya seeds

Water to thin as necessary

Put papaya, avocado, lemon juice and vinegar in the blender. Blend until smooth, adding water to thin if necessary. Add the basil, pinch of salt, and optional oil and papaya seeds. The oil will make the dressing creamier and less perishable. You also don't have to use a full tablespoon. The papaya seeds impart a peppery taste—a little goes a long way, so try a small amount of seeds first! Pulse in these remaining ingredients. Great over a simple romaine-tomato salad with some soaked sea veggies.

Ranch Dressing

1 ¼ cup sunflower seeds

3 celery ribs

½ cup + 2 Tablespoons lemon juice

1 clove garlic, optional

2 Tablespoon raw tahini

1 teaspoon Celtic sea salt, optional

½ teaspoon onion powder

1¾ cup purified water

¾ teaspoon basil

½ teaspoon oregano

½ teaspoon thyme

kelp, dulse and/or celery powder to taste

Presoak sunflower seeds for at least 6 hours. Blend the first eight ingredients until smooth. Add the basil, oregano and thyme, and favorite seasonings to taste into the blender, and blend on low speed for five seconds. Pour the dressing onto grated vegetables (e.g. carrots, cabbage, zucchini) and toss to coat. Serve.

Cooked Recipes

Lemon-Braised Spinach in Coconut Milk

Remember we said that it's good to eat greens with some fat, in order to absorb the fat-soluble vitamins? And we said coconut is very stable under heat? As well as being so delicious, this recipe combines those two good insights.

Serves 2-4

1 medium onion, chopped

1 pound spinach

1 tablespoon ginger, grated

2 tablespoons lemon juice

zest of one lemon

1 14-oz can coconut milk (look for a brand with no added preservatives.)

1 teaspoon sea salt, or to taste

1 teaspoon garlic powder, optional

Cilantro leaves, for garnishing

Heat a heavy-bottomed skillet. When it is hot, add the onion with a little water, and sauté until the onion is partially cooked, about five minutes. Add the ginger and lemon zest, and cook for a couple more minutes.

Add the spinach to the pan. You'll need to do this a handful at a time—wait for what's in the pan to wilt down before adding more.

Once all the spinach is in the pan, add the coconut milk, lemon juice, and garlic powder and salt, if using.

Let simmer for ten minutes.

Garnish with chopped cilantro just before serving. This is great over sweet potatoes or other cooked starches.

Vegan Penang Curry

The hallmark of Thai-style curries called "Penang" or "Massaman" is the inclusion of peanuts and/or peanut butter. The coconut base protects the polyunsaturated fats in the peanut butter from the heat of cooking. The tofu is optional, but if you choose to include it, the dish will be even higher in fat overall, and very rich in general.

Serves 2-6

1 small onion, finely chopped

1 tablespoon ginger, grated

2 tablespoons galangal (Thai ginger), grated *if you can find it; if not, just use more ginger*

2 cloves garlic, minced

2 teaspoons turmeric

2 teaspoons ground coriander

1 tablespoon curry powder

¼ cup peanut butter

1 cup water

1 14-oz can coconut milk (look for a brand with no added preservatives.)

1 tablespoon maple syrup

1 teaspoon sea salt, optional

1 sweet potato, peeled and cut into chunks

4 cups Napa cabbage, torn into pieces (or other green of choice)

1-2 carrots, cut into matchsticks

1 can bamboo shoots

Optional: 1 14-oz package extra-firm tofu, soaked, rinsed, drained and cut into bite-sized pieces (If you freeze the tofu first, it will drain even more, which will make it absorb the flavors and liquids of the curry even better.)

Thai basil, for garnishing (Use regular basil, or cilantro, if you can't find Thai basil.)

Heat a large, heavy-bottomed pan and add the onion, garlic, and gingers, with a little water. Cook until softened, about five minutes.

Add the turmeric, coriander, curry powder, and peanut butter. Cook a couple more minutes, stirring continuously.

Mix in the water, coconut milk, maple syrup, and salt.

When these are all incorporated, add the vegetables, and the tofu if using, and bring to a boil.

Cover, and simmer until everything is tender, about 30 minutes.

Check for seasonings—possibly add a little lemon juice or cayenne pepper.

Serve garnished with Thai basil.

Leek and Sweet Potato Bisque

Serves 6-8

3 cups medium sweet potatoes

3 large leeks, white and light-green parts only

1 quart unsweetened almond milk, or more

2 cups water

1 tablespoon grated ginger

½ teaspoon onion powder

½ teaspoon white pepper

1 teaspoon kelp powder

stevia to taste

Cut each sweet potato in half, and bake in a 350 degree oven until tender, 40 minutes to an hour.

Meanwhile, trim and clean the leeks thoroughly. Slice lengthwise and rinse well, taking care to remove the grit that may have accumulated between the layers. Slice into half-inch semicircles.

Put the leeks in a large stockpot with the grated ginger, cover, and cook for about five minutes, stirring occasionally and adding a little water if necessary.

Turn the heat down and keep cooking the leeks for another 20 minutes, stirring occasionally and adding a little water as needed.

Take the pot off the heat and add the flesh (not the skin) of the sweet potatoes.

Add the almond milk and the seasonings.

Using an immersion blender, puree until everything is smooth, or leave it slightly chunky if you prefer. Add more water or almond milk as necessary to achieve your desired texture. (If you don't have an immersion blender, you can get the same result, but with more associated cleanup, by pureeing in batches in a regular blender, making sure to fill it no more than halfway since your soup is hot.)

Kale Veggie Stew

This hearty stew contains plenty of legumes, a great source of protein and complex carbs, together with mushrooms and onions, both highly prized for their cancer-fighting compounds. It also models the advice to cook some greens into your stews as a great way to keep getting more greens in. Plus, this dish contains no fat except what is in the beans and vegetables, a very small quantity!

Serves 2-4

½ **cup** cooked red kidney beans

1 ¼ **cup** mixed dry beans and lentils; soaked 12 hours

8 **cups** water

1 **800ml can** tomatoes

2 **cans** small sweet peas (divided use)

4 **ribs** celery, chopped

2 medium yellow onions, chopped

4 large carrots diced or grated

1 **whole head** garlic, minced

8 large mushrooms, finely chopped

1 large bay leaf

1 tablespoon dried rosemary

1 tablespoon thyme

1 tablespoon turmeric

1 bunch kale, washed, de-stemmed, and finely chopped

parsley leaves, for garnishing

pinches of salt and pepper, to taste

Drain the soaked beans and boil in a large stockpot with 8 cups cold water for 45 minutes.

Then add the tomatoes, one can of peas, celery, onion, carrot, garlic, mushrooms, and seasonings.

Cover and cook for another half hour (or until beans and veggies are tender). Add the chopped kale, and cook 20 minutes more.

Put half of the stew in the blender and blend thoroughly before returning to the pot. Alternatively, use an immersion blender to puree the stew partially.

Stir in the second can of peas.

Serve garnished with fresh parsley.

This is a good recipe to make on the weekend and freeze in portioned containers so you're set for the week!

Indian Dal

This is a recipe I make quite often, at least 3-4 times a month. It's so easy to make, and can be customized once you have the basic recipe mastered.

6 cups vegetable stock or water

1 1/2 cups red lentils (rinsed)

3-4 cloves garlic

1 teaspoon cumin powder

cayenne powder **to taste**

1 teaspoon turmeric

1/4 teaspoon cardamom

2-3 bay leaves

2 teaspoon mustard seeds

Traditionally, you would sauté the garlic in oil before adding in the other spices. Spices can be toasted for more flavor. I personally dump everything in a non-stick cooking pot.

Bring to a boil. Then lower heat and simmer for 35 minutes or so.

Variations: add a few diced tomatoes, fresh or canned.

Sesame-Seared Tuna

This is a recipe for nearly raw fish. Get the highest-quality tuna you can find. White or red tuna is great for this recipe.

1/8 cup dark soy sauce

1/8 cup light soy sauce

1 tablespoon mirin (Japanese sweet wine)

1 tablespoon maple syrup or honey

1 tablespoon toasted sesame oil

1 tablespoon rice wine vinegar

1/2 cup sesame seeds

wasabi paste

a bit of oil to coat pan (you can alternatively try it dry on a hot pan).

3-4 tuna steaks of about **6 ounces** each

1- In a bowl make a marinade with the soy sauce, mirin, maple syrup or honey, and sesame oil. Keep 1/3 to 1/2 of this sauce apart as a dipping sauce, in a separate bowl. Mix in the rice vinegar for this dipping sauce.

Let the tuna marinate for a few minutes in the sauce. Spread sesame seeds on a plate, and coat the tuna steaks with them by pressing them on the plate where the sesame seeds rest.

Heat a pan until very hot, add a tiny bit of oil, and sear steaks for about 30 seconds each side. Should be rare inside (can also be cooked thoroughly if you prefer, but flavor is lost).

Serve with dipping sauce and wasabi.

Marinated Wild Salmon

1/4 cup capers

1/4 white mellow miso

1/8 cup olive oil

2 tablespoon maple syrup

1/2 cup mirin

Around **2 pounds** wild salmon fillets

Crush the capers with a fork, and mix with the other ingredients to create a sauce. Let the salmon fillets marinate in this sauce by placing them inside a sealable plastic bag with the sauce for about one hour (or longer) in the refrigerator.

Cook in a preheated 425-degree oven for 15 to 20 minutes on a baking sheet. Alternatively, for a healthier version, the fillets can be steamed and the remaining sauce served on top of them.

Easy Black Beans

I love black beans, so I usually make a batch every couple of weeks. With my method, you won't need to soak the beans in advance

2 cups dried black beans

2 cloves garlic (peeled, but whole)

1 small potato, peeled

2 bay leaves

Sea salt **to taste**

Rinse the beans in a colander, and then sort through them to remove any rocks or overly dried, broken, or shriveled beans. If you buy good quality black beans, there should not be too many broken beans.

Put in a pot with all the other ingredients, and add enough water to cover them, leaving 2-3 inches of water on top. Bring to a boil, and then reduce heat to the lowest setting possible. Cover, and let it cook for about two hours, or until the beans are soft to your liking. Then season with salt (usually a good amount, because most of it will be lost in the water). Discard the potato, bay leaves, and garlic cloves.

Cooked beans will keep for 4-5 days in the fridge.

Hummus

2 cups cooked chickpeas (or use a 16-oz can)

1/4 cup liquid from cooking, or from the can

3-5 tablespoons lemon juice (to taste)

1 1/2 tablespoons tahini

2 cloves garlic, crushed (can use less)

1/2 teaspoon salt

1/2 teaspoon cumin

Put all ingredients in a food processor fitted with the S-blade. Puree until completely smooth, adding more liquid if necessary (this can be more lemon juice or more chickpea water; traditionally, some olive oil gets drizzled in. If you're cooking the chickpeas yourself, interestingly, you'll get better results if you work with warm chickpeas!

Serve garnished with paprika and capers.

Babaghanoush

Babaghanoush is sort of like hummus with smoky eggplant instead of chickpeas. It is just one name for a dip ubiquitous all over the Middle East.

1 large eggplant

1/4 cup lemon juice

1/4 cup tahini

2 cloves garlic, minced

salt and pepper **to taste**

It's best to go by taste because each eggplant is different and will cook differently. Traditionally, the eggplant is fire-roasted over an open flame, but doing it this way is often impractical.

Baking the eggplant in a small oven is best, and results in the best flavor. Make sure to poke holes in it first so it doesn't explode in the oven. Preheat the oven to 400 degrees F (200 Celsius), and then bake for at least 40 minutes, turning once. It should be fully cooked. Put it in cold water, and then peel the skin off. Wait until it cools.

You have to be careful with the eggplant liquid. Drain the liquid, but save it in case you need it.

Place the peeled eggplant in a food processor or blender with the rest of the ingredients, and blend. Use eggplant liquid if you need it to achieve the right consistency. Make sure to season to taste.

Ratatouille

This is a traditional French stew based on onions and tomatoes. Hearty, red, delicious.

2 tablespoons olive oil (optional)

2 cloves garlic, minced

1 large onion, chopped

1 small or medium eggplant, cubed

2 green bell peppers, diced

4 large tomatoes, coarsely chopped, or **2 cans (14.5 ounces each)** diced tomatoes

3 to 4 small zucchini, cut into 1/4-inch slices

1 teaspoon Herbes de Provence mix

salt and pepper **to taste**

Sauté the onion and garlic in the olive oil, if using. Otherwise, steam-sauté with a little water.

After about five minutes, add the eggplant and cook for another 8-10 minutes.

Then add the remaining vegetables, cover, and let the liquid from the tomatoes cook everything together and reduce down to a delicious stew.

Butternut Squash Chowder

Serves 4-5

4 cups vegetable broth or water

1 large onion, diced

5 cloves garlic, minced

6 cups butternut squash, peeled and cubed (fresh or frozen)

2 1/2 cups sweet corn (fresh, frozen or canned – no sodium)

1 16 oz. can white beans, drained

1/2 teaspoon smoked paprika (or any other seasoning of choice)

3/4 teaspoon Herbamare or salt

1/2 teaspoon freshly ground pepper

Directions:

Sauté onions and garlic in a large pot over medium heat in 1/2 cup of vegetable broth until soft 5-6 minutes.

Add squash, corn and beans, and remaining broth, and cover. Cook until squash is tender.

Carefully spoon mixture into a blender or food processor and blend until smooth, or use an immersion blender and puree in the pot.

Pour mixture back into pot, add seasonings and mix thoroughly. Taste test and adjust seasonings if desired.

Black Bean Soup

Another hearty staple you should have in your rotation.

1 red onion, diced

6 cloves garlic, minced

1 teaspoon cumin

2 teaspoons chili powder

dash cinnamon, salt

2 tablespoons sucanat (unrefined cane sugar)

6 tomatoes, chopped (or use **2 cans** roasted tomatoes)

3 cans black beans, drained (or **6 cups** home-cooked beans)

5 cups vegetable stock

1 bunch cilantro, chopped

juice of **one** lime (or at least **2 tablespoons**)

Method

Steam-sauté the onion and garlic in a heated, heavy bottomed stockpot, with a little water as necessary until well softened, about 5 minutes.

Add the spices and sucanat, and cook another 2-3 minutes.

Add the rest of the ingredients to the pot, except for the cilantro and lime juice.

Cook for 20-30 minutes, until everything is well combined and the liquids reduced so that the soup is not watery. Add the cilantro and lime juice, and adjust seasonings to taste.

Made in the USA
Charleston, SC
08 April 2013